Microbiology
PreTest® Self-Assessment and Review

Notice

Medicine is an ever-changing science. As new research and clinical experience broaden our knowledge, changes in treatment and drug therapy are required. The authors and the publisher of this work have checked with sources believed to be reliable in their efforts to provide information that is complete and generally in accord with the standards accepted at the time of publication. However, in view of the possibility of human error or changes in medical sciences, neither the authors nor the publisher nor any other party who has been involved in the preparation or publication of this work warrants that the information contained herein is in every respect accurate or complete, and they disclaim all responsibility for any errors or omissions or for the results obtained from use of the information contained in this work. Readers are encouraged to confirm the information contained herein with other sources. For example and in particular, readers are advised to check the product information sheet included in the package of each drug they plan to administer to be certain that the information contained in this work is accurate and that changes have not been made in the recommended dose or in the contraindications for administration. This recommendation is of particular importance in connection with new or infrequently used drugs.

Microbiology
PreTest® Self-Assessment and Review
Eleventh Edition

James D. Kettering, Ph.D.
Professor of Microbiology and Associate Chairman—Microbiology
Department of Biochemistry and Microbiology
Loma Linda University
School of Medicine
Loma Linda, California

Craig A. Seheult, M.S. (Microbiology)
Contributor—Immunology and Physiology/Molecular Microbiology
Loma Linda University
School of Medicine
Loma Linda, California
Class of 2007

McGraw-Hill
Medical Publishing Division
New York   Chicago   San Francisco   Lisbon   London   Madrid   Mexico City
Milan   New Delhi   San Juan   Seoul   Singapore   Sydney   Toronto

The **McGraw·Hill** Companies

Microbiology: PreTest® Self-Assessment and Review, Eleventh Edition

1 2 3 4 5 6 7 8 9 0 DOC/DOC 0 9 8 7 6 5 4

ISBN 0-07-143748-7

This book was set in Berkeley by North Market Street Graphics.
The editor was Catherine A. Johnson.
The production supervisor was Phil Galea.
Project management was provided by North Market Street Graphics.
The cover designer was Li Chen Chang / Pinpoint.
RR Donnelley was printer and binder.

This book is printed on acid-free paper.

Cataloging-in-Publication data is on file for this title at the Library of Congress.

Student Reviewers

Frances Ford
Eastern Carolina University Brody School of Medicine
Greenville, North Carolina
Class of 2004

Sarah Harper
University of Pittsburgh School of Medicine
Pittsburgh, Pennsylvania
Class of 2005

Alisa A. Meny
UMDNJ—Robert Wood Johnson Medical School
Piscataway, New Jersey
Class of 2004

Sabara Nandi
UMDNJ—Robert Wood Johnson Medical School
Piscataway, New Jersey
Class of 2003

Adam J. Rosh
UMDNJ—Robert Wood Johnson Medical School
Piscataway, New Jersey
Class of 2004

Contents

Introduction ix
Acknowledgments x

High-Yield Facts

High-Yield Facts in Microbiology I

Physiology and Molecular Microbiology

Questions 15
Answers 36

Virology

Questions 49
Answers 79

Bacteriology

Questions 107
Answers 141

Rickettsiae, Chlamydiae, and Mycoplasmas

Questions 173
Answers 182

Mycology

Questions 189
Answers 203

Parasitology

Questions 213
Answers 233

Immunology

Questions 245
Answers 278

Bibliography 303
Index 305

Introduction

Each *PreTest® Self-Assessment and Review* allows medical students to comprehensively and conveniently assess and review their knowledge of a particular basic science, in this instance microbiology. The 500 questions parallel the format and degree of difficulty of the questions found in the United States Medical Licensing Examination (USMLE) Step 1. Practicing physicians who want to hone their skills before USMLE Step 3 or recertification may find this to be a good beginning in their review process. Each question is accompanied by an answer, a paragraph explanation, and a specific page reference to an appropriate textbook or journal article. A bibliography listing sources can be found following the last chapter of this text.

An effective way to use this PreTest® is to allow yourself one minute to answer each question in a given chapter. As you proceed, indicate your answer beside each question. By following this suggestion, you approximate the time limits imposed by the Step 1 exam.

After you finish going through the questions in the section, spend as much time as you need verifying your answers and carefully reading the explanations provided. Pay special attention to the explanations for the questions you answered incorrectly, but read every explanation. The authors of this material have designed the explanations to reinforce and supplement the information tested by the questions. If you feel you need further information about the material covered, consult and study the references indicated.

The High-Yield Facts added for this edition are provided to facilitate rapid review of microbiology. It is anticipated that the reader will use the High-Yield Facts as a "memory jog" before proceeding through the questions.

Acknowledgments

The author wishes to thank Raydolfo M. Aprecio, O.D., and David E. Kettering, J.D., for expert assistance in the production of the manuscript for this revision.

High-Yield Facts

PHYSIOLOGY AND MOLECULAR BIOLOGY

- Koch's postulates: (1) Specific organism must be in diseased animal; (2) organism must be isolated in pure culture; (3) organism produces disease in healthy susceptible animal; (4) organism reisolated from infected animal.
- Gram stain: (1) Fixation; (2) crystal violet; (3) iodine treatment; (4) decolorization (alcohol/acetone); (5) counterstain (safranin). Gram-positive = purple; gram-negative = red.
- Gram stain poor for: *Chlamydia, Mycoplasma, Rickettsia, Treponema, Mycobacteria* (use acid-fast stain), *Legionella* (use silver stain).
- Bacterial shapes: Bacilli (rod), cocci (spherical), spirilla (spiral), square, and filamentous.
- Bacterial aggregates: Diplococci (e.g., Neisseriae), Streptococci (chains), tetrads (fours), Staphylococci (clusters), Sarcinae (cubes).
- Flagella: Monotrichous—single polar flagellum; lophotrichous—cluster of flagella at pole; amphitrichous—flagella at both poles; peritrichous—flagella encircling the cell.
- Type VII pili = F or sex pili; important in bacterial conjugation.
- Conjugation—DNA transferred from one bacterium to another; transduction—viral transfer of DNA from one cell to another; transformation—cellular uptake of purified DNA.
- Peptidoglycan (murein or mucopeptide) layer: unique to prokaryotes, consist of glycan polymers of sugar N-acetylglucosamine (NAG) and N-acetylmuramic acid (NAM) and cross-linked by a short peptide. Cross-linking enzymes are transpeptidases (targets for β-lactam antibiotics).
- Bacterial structures: Peptidoglycan (support); cell wall/membrane (antigenic); outer membrane (LPS/endotoxin); plasma membrane (oxidative/transport enzymes); ribosome (protein synthesis); periplasmic space (hydrolytic enzymes and β-lactamases); capsule (antiphagocytic, polysaccharide except *Bacillus anthracis*, which is D-glutamate); pilus/fimbria (adherence, conjugation); flagellum (motility); spore (heat, chemical, dehydration resistance, consists of dipicolinic acid); plasmid (genes for toxins, enzymes, antibiotic resistance); glycocalyx (adherence, made of polysaccharide); inclusion bodies (no membrane; store glycogen, polyphosphate, poly-β-hydroxybutyric acid).
- Gram-positive: Teichoic acid unique.
- Gram-negative: Lipopolysaccharide (LPS; endotoxin) unique.
- LPS (endotoxin): Lipid A covalently linked to polysaccharide core and then unique "D antigen" polysaccharide repeat; illicits acute-phase protein response in vivo (release of TNF-α, IL-1, IL-6) causing fever, etc.
- Lysozyme: Breaks down glycan backbone bonds of peptidoglycan (β1-4 bonds between NAM and NAG).

I

- Spheroplast: Partial cell-wall lysozyme digestion.
- Protoplast: Complete cell-wall lysozyme digestion.
- Geometric growth: Cell number = $a(2^n)$, where a is number of starting cells, n equals number of generations.
- Bacterial growth curves (four phases): (1) Lag (no cellular division, cell size increase); (2) exponential (regular doubling time, essential nutrients decrease, toxins increase); (3) stationary (cell division rate = cell death rate); (4) death (cell energy stores depleted, exponential death to low population equilibrium).
- Bacteriostatic: Agent inhibits multiplication, growth resumes upon removal of agent.
- Bactericidal: Agent kills bacteria, irreversible.
- Sterile: Free from all forms of life.
- Disinfectant: Chemical kills bacteria but toxic to tissue.
- Septic: Pathogenic organism present in living tissue.
- Aseptic: Pathogenic organism not present in living tissue.
- Passive transport: No energy, movement down concentration gradient, no carrier molecule.
- Active transport: Requires energy, against concentration gradient.
- Fluoride ion (water, toothpaste, etc.): Inhibits several cellular bacterial enzymes, especially enolase.
- Bacterial pathogenesis: (1) Antiphagocytic (cell-wall proteins—protein A in *Staphylococcus aureus* and protein M in *Streptococcus pyogenes,* capsules, pili/fimbriae); (2) adherence factors (pili/fimbriae, lipoteichoic acid, glycocalyx, adhesion); (3) enzymes (coagulase, collagenase, fibrinolysin, hyaluronidase, lecithinase, mucinase); (4) toxins (exotoxins, endotoxins/LPS).
- Exotoxins: Polypeptide, highly fatal, toxoids as vaccines, heat labile, secreted, both gram-negative and gram-positive.
- Endotoxins: Lipopolysaccharide, low toxicity, no toxoids, no vaccines, heat stable, released on lysis, only gram-negative.
- Free radicals of oxygen (superoxides) kill anaerobic bacteria exposed to air. Superoxide dismutase is a potent bacterial antioxidant. The perixodases in bacteria are protective.
- Obligate anaerobes: Lack catalase and/or superoxide dismutase and susceptible to oxidative damage, foul smelling, produce gas in tissue (e.g., *Actinomyces, Bacteroides,* and *Clostridium*).
- Superoxide dismutase catalyzes: $2O_2^- + 2H^+ \rightarrow H_2O_2 + O_2$
- Catalase catalyzes: $2H_2O_2 \rightarrow 2H_2O + O_2$
- Myeloperoxidase catalyzes: $Cl^- + H_2O_2 \rightarrow ClO^- + H_2O$
- NADPH oxidase catalyzes: $NADPH + 2O_2 \rightarrow 2O_2^- + H^+ NADP^+$
- Sites of action of antimicrobial agents include cell-wall synthesis, cell-membrane integrity, DNA replication, protein synthesis, DNA-dependent RNA polymerase, folic acid metabolism.

VIROLOGY

Virus basics—terms: virion, capsid, capsomere, nucleocapsid
- All DNA viruses are ds, except Parvovirus.
- All DNA viruses have linear DNA, except papovaviruses and hepadnaviruses.
- All RNA viruses have ssRNA, except reoviruses.
- Segmented RNA viruses include orthomyxoviruses and reoviruses.
- Positive sense RNA (same as mRNA) include picornaviruses, and caliciviruses, Flaviviruses, retroviruses, and coronaviruses. All other RNA viruses are negative sense (need viral RNA polymerase).
- Obligate intracellular parasites, using viral receptors to attach to host cell receptors.
- Growth cycle: Attachment, entry, eclipse, maturation, release.
- Viral disease patterns: Acute, chronic, latent (persistent).
- DNA viruses grow in the host nucleus (except poxviruses).
- RNA viruses grow in the host cytoplasm (except influenza and retroviruses).

Hepatitis Viruses
- Hepatitis A (HAV)—Picornavirus, fecal oral transmission, no chronic carriers.
- Hepatitis B (HBV)—Hepadnavirus, parental, sexual transmission passes through placenta, acute and chronic disease, HBV possesses a reverse transcriptase polymerase.
- Hepatitis C (HCV)—Flavivirus, +ssRNA, parental, sexual transmission, acute and chronic disease.
- Hepatitis D (HDV)—"Delta" hepatitis—defective virus, requires HBV coinfection, acute and chronic infections.
- Hepatitis E (HEV)—Calicivirus, +ssRNA, fecal-oral transmission.

HAV and HBV have approved vaccines.

DNA Viruses
- Parvovirus B19—ssDNA—causes fifth disease/erythema infectiosum (slapped cheek appearance).
- Papovaviruses.
  - Papillomaviruses—ds circular DNA—cause warts (HPV type 1, 4—benign; 6, 11—anogenital; 16, 18—cervical carcinoma).
  - Polyoma viruses—BK—kidney disease; JC (progressive multifocal leukoencepalopathy).
- Adenovirus (ds linear DNA)—conjunctivitis and respiratory diseases in kids. Strains 10, 41 cause gastroenteritis.
- Herpesviruses.
  - Herpes simplex—latent infections common.
  - HSV-1—trigeminal ganglia; cold sores, conjunctivitis, and encephalitis (treat with acyclovir).

- HSV-2—sacral nerve ganglia—sexually transmitted.
- Varicella—zoster—chickenpox-shingles—lesions are asynchronous (all forms present). Vaccine attenuated.
- Cytomegalovirus—common; direct and sexual contact for transmission; retinitis and pneumonitis in immunocompromised; neonates—CMV inclusion disease.
- Epstein-Barr virus—infects B lymphocytes; causes infectious mononucleosis; positive for heterophile antibodies—EBV—EA (early antigen), VCA (viral capsid antigen), EBNA (nuclear antigen)—diagnostic value.
- Poxviruses—large, dsDNA—grow in cytoplasm, complex envelope.
  - Variola—smallpox, extinct since 1977. Bioterrorism agent. Vaccinia virus—vaccine strain.
  - Molluscum contagiosum—benign tumors.

Positive ssRNA Viruses
- Picornavirus (+ssRNA).
  - Polio, coxsackie A and B, echoviruses, HAV—polio—Salk/Sabin vaccines; U.S. now uses killed vaccine.
  - All strains cause upper respiratory infections (URIs), rashes, limited central nervous system (CNS) infections (glucose normal; protein—elevated slightly); gastrointestinal (GI), hemorrhagic conjunctivitis, and myocarditis.
- Rhinoviruses—common cold.
  - Flaviviruses—HCV, yellow fever, dengue, Saint Louis encephalitis.
  - Togaviruses—Western Equine encephalitis, Eastern Equine encephalitis, Venezuelan Equine encephalitis, West Nile virus (birds and horses—normal hosts).
  - Rubella virus—German measles—(no insect vector)—causes severe birth defects.
  - Coronaviruses—common cold mostly; also severe acute respiratory syndrome (SARS).
  - Retroviruses—diploid genome—gag genes—p24, p7, p9, and p17; env—gp 120 and gp 41; pol gene reverse transcriptase/integrase; progene-protease AIDS (CD4) <200 lymphocytes/mm^3. Opportunistic infections—*Candida, Mycobacterium* species, multiple viruses, and protozoan.

Negative ssRNA viruses
- Require virion-associated RNA-dependent RNA polymerase.
- Paramyxoviruses.
- Measles—fever, conjunctivitis, Koplic's spots—rash.
- Complications—pneumonia, encephalitis; good vaccine.
- Mumps—salivary, parotid glands; orchitis; good liver vaccine.
- Respiratory syncytial virus—major cause of URI—infants (treat with ribovirin).

- Rhabdovirus—bullet-shaped—U.S. reservoirs—skunks, raccoons, foxes, coyotes/dogs, and bats; animal bite transmission; control animal vectors; Negri body—eosinophilic intracytoplasmic inclusion body.
- Orthomyxoviruses.
- Influenza A and B, segmented genomes.
- Genetic drift—minor antigen changes; genetic shift—major new hemagglutinin and/or neuraminidase changes.
- Bunyaviruses—California encephalitis virus; hantavirus.
- Arenaviruses—lymphocytic choriomenigitis virus, Lassa fever.

dsRNA Viruses—Double-Shelled Capsids.
- Rotaviruses—infantile diarrhea.
- Reoviruses—common in humans, febrile diseases.

BACTERIOLOGY

- Gram-positive cocci: Staphylococci catalase +, Streptococci catalase −.
- *S. aureus:* Mannitol-salt agar (selective and differential), yellow colonies, coagulase +, mannitol +, catalase +, methicillin resistant, some vancomycin resistance emerging, protein A (binds IgG Fc inhibiting phagocytosis), rapid-onset food poisoning (enterotoxin), toxic shock syndrome, scalded skin syndrome, osteomyelitis, acute bacterial endocarditis (IV drug users), abscesses, recurrent infection in chronic granulomatous disease (CGD).
- Streptococci: β-hemolytic divided into groups (13 groups: A–O) based on cell-wall carbohydrate antigens. Group A divided into ≥50 types based on M proteins (virulence, specific immunity), catalase−.
- *S. pyogenes* (group A): Hyaluronic acid capsule, carbohydrate antigen, M protein, bacitracin sensitive, cellulitis, rheumatic fever, glomerulonephritis, necrotizing fasciitis, erysipelas, scarlet fever.
- *Streptococcus viridans:* Normal oral flora, α-hemolytic, subacute bacterial endocarditis after dental/oral surgery.
- *Streptococcus faecalis* (group D): Normal intestinal flora, subacute bacterial endocarditis after pelvic/abdominal surgery, urinary tract infections (UTIs), growth in 6.5% NaCl.
- *Streptococcus agalactiae* (group B): Normal vaginal flora; in dairy products (cattle pathogen); neonatal sepsis; Christie, Atkins, Munch-Peterson (CAMP) test+.
- Peptostreptococci: Normal oral/vaginal flora, endocarditis, lung abscess.
- *Streptococcus pneumoniae:* Pneumonia, meningitis, otitis media (children), optochin sensitive, bile soluble, use quellung reaction, pneumococcal polyvalent vaccine.
- Dick test: Test susceptibility to scarlet fever.
- Shultz-Charlton test: Determine if rash is due to erythrogenic toxin of scarlet fever.

- Gram-negative cocci (*Neisseria*): Oxidase +, diplococci, polysaccharide capsule, associated with C5, 6, 7, 8 complement deficiency; pathogenic forms: Thayer-Martin agar +, chocolate agar +, nutrient agar −, 37°C growth +, room temperature −; nonpathogenic forms: Thayer-Martin agar −, chocolate agar +, nutrient agar +, 37°C growth +, room temperature +.
- *Neisseria menigitidis:* Capsule, endotoxin, toxemia, petechiae, hemorrhage, disseminated intravascular coagulation (DIC).
- Bacterial meningitis in <40-year-old = *N. meningitidis;* >40-year-old = *S. pneumoniae;* 2–60 months = *Haemophilus influenzae.*
- *Neisseria gonorrhoeae:* Pili, IgA protease, pharyngitis, proctitis, pelvic inflammatory disease (PID), urethritis, cervicitis.
- Gram-positive Bacilli: Aerobic (Bacilli); anaerobic (*Clostridium*), killed by autoclave.
- *B. anthracis:* Polypeptide capsule, exotoxin, anthrax (wool-sorters' disease).
- *Bacillus cereus:* Food poisoning, enterotoxin.
- *Clostridium:* No cytochrome enzymes, no catalase, no superoxide dismutase.
- *Clostridium tetani:* Noninvasive, neurotoxins (prevents release of neural inhibitory transmitters such as γ-aminobutyric acid [GABA] and glycine), lockjaw, give toxoid/antitoxin.
- *Clostridium botulinum:* Noninvasive, exotoxins (prevents acetylcholine release), flaccid paralysis, antitoxin.
- *Clostridium perfringens:* Invasive, enterotoxin, food poisoning, myonecrosis, collagenase, lecithinase, gas gangrene.
- *Clostridium difficile:* Pseudomembranous colitis, can occur after broad-spectrum antibiotic usage.
- *Corynebacterium diphtheria:* Gram-positive rod, metachromatic granules, exotoxin (inhibits EF-2 and protein synthesis).
- *Listeria monocytogenes:* Gram+ rod in cerebrospinal fluid (CSF), compromised host, neonate, diarrhea after eating raw cheeses.
- *Salmonella:* Gram-negative rod, enteric fever, food poisoning; *Salmonella typhi* = human pathogen; other species = animal pathogens; motile; nonlactose fermenter.
- *Shigella:* Gram-negative rod, more virulent than *Salmonella,* bloody diarrhea, shigellosis is human disease, oral-anal route, toxin inhibits protein synthesis.
- *Escherichia coli:* Gram-negative rod, most common UTI infection, sepsis (serious); EHEC (colitis, hemolytic uremic syndrome-verotoxin, hamburger, beef); EIEC (fever, bloody stool, diarrhea); ETEC (traveler's diarrhea); EPEC (infant fever and diarrhea, nonbloody stool).
- *Pseudomonas aeruginosa:* Gram-negative rod, antibiotic resistance, pigments, UTI, wounds, burns.
- *Klebsiella:* Large capsule, UTI, pneumonia.
- *H. influenzae:* Gram-negative rod, meningitis, otitis, sinusitis, epiglottitis.
- *Proteus:* Gram-negative rod, urease (urea → NH_3)—also produced by *Helicobacter pylori* and *Ureaplasma urealyticum;* UTI, wounds, renal stones.

- *Gardnerella vaginalis:* "Clue cells"; vaginitis with discharge (fishy smell).
- *Bordetella pertussis:* Capsule, pili, killed vaccine, whooping cough.
- *Yersinia pestis:* "Safety pin" (bipolar staining), plague (bubonic/pneumonic), rat flea.
- *Francisella tularensis:* Skinning rabbits (jackrabbits), tularemia.
- *Pasteurella multocida:* Cat/dog bites; cellulitis, "shipping fever."
- *Brucella:* Dye sensitivity test, undulent fever.
- *Mycobacterium tuberculosis:* Tuberculosis, acid-fast stain, Lowenstein-Jensen medium.
- *Mycobacterium leprae:* Leprosy, cannot be cultured.
- *Haemophilus ducreyi:* Painful lesion, chancroid (syphilis: painless chancre).
- *Treponema pallidum:* VDRL, FTA/ABS, IgM antibody, use penicillin G, three stages, spirochetes, dark-field microscopy.
- *Borrelia:* Aniline dyes (Wright's/Giemsa), *Ixodes* tick, relapsing fever, Lyme disease, acute necrotizing ulcerative gingivitis.
- *Legionella pneumophila:* Legionnaires' disease, fulminating pneumonia, gramnegative rod, airborne through contaminated water (air-conditioner cooling system).
- Exotoxin: Heat labile.
- Endotoxin (LPS): Heat stable.
- Diphtheria/*Pseudomonas* exotoxin: Act via ADP-ribosylation of EF-2, thus protein synthesis inhibited.
- *E. coli, Vibrio cholerae, B. cereus* heat-labile enterotoxin: ADP-ribosylation of G_s protein turns G_s protein on, thus activating adenylate cyclase, leading to ↑cAMP and diarrhea.
- *B. pertussis* heat-labile enterotoxin: ADP-ribosylation of G_i protein turns off G_i protein, thereby activating adenylate cyclase, leading to ↑cAMP and diarrhea.
- *Vibrio:* Oxidase positive; one flagellum; curved, "comma-shaped" gram-negative rod; halophilic (except *V. cholerae*).
- *Vibrio parahaemolyticus:* Contaminated seafood, diarrhea.
- *Vibrio vulnificus:* Contaminated marine animals (oyster ingestion), diarrhea, skin lesions (handling).
- Vancomycin-resistant enterococci, methicillin-resistant *S. aureus* (MRSA), and vancomycin-indeterminate *S. aureus* (VISA) are among the most feared nosocomial pathogens. A recently introduced antibiotic, quinapristin-delfapristin, effectively treats vancomycin-resistant enterococci or the few vancomycin-indeterminate MRSAs that have occurred.
- Following an upsurge of tuberculosis in the early 1990s, cases of *M. tuberculosis* infection have remained static. *M. tuberculosis* causes initial primary pulmonary infection as well as a chronic disease characterized by hemoptysis, loss of weight, and fever.
- Penicillin-resistant pneumococci (*S. pneumoniae*) may account for up to 40% of isolates of *S. pneumoniae*. Third- or fourth-generation cephalosporins may be used as alternative treatment as well as vancomycin and rifampin.

- *Campylobacter* and *Helicobacter* are both helical-shaped bacteria. *Helicobacter* is known to play a role in the pathogenesis of peptic ulcer disease, while *Campylobacter* causes a food-borne gastrointestinal illness, most commonly from undercooked meat. Both bacteria are susceptible to antibiotics such as tetracycline. *Helicobacter* may be treated with Pepto-Bismol, metronidazole, and amoxicillin.

RICKETTSIAE, CHLAMYDIAE, MYCOPLASMAS

Rickettsiae

- *Rickettsia, Coxiella, Bartonella (Rochalimaea)*, and *Ehrlichia*—main genera. All are obligate intracellular parasites due to limited ATP production. Insect vectors include ticks, mites, body lice.
- Rocky Mountain spotted fever—*Rickettsia rickettsii*—spread by ticks, invades capillaries, causing vasculitis. Rash commonly moves from extremities to trunk. Diagnosis is usually serology, using cross-reacting antibodies to *P. vulgaris* OX strains.
- Treat with tetracyclines.
- *Coxiella burnetii*—reservoir is livestock; inhalation transmission. Causes Q fever, an atypical pneumonia.
- *Bartonella*—pericellular, not intracellular infection. (*Bartonella quintana, Bartonella henselae*) Causes trench fever, septicemia, cat-scratch disease.
- *Ehrlichia*—infects monocytes, granulocytes; tick transmission.

Chlamydiae

- Obligate intracellular parasites that do not produce ATP. Possess a modified gram-negative cell wall. A true bacterium.
- Unusual life cycle—infectious elementary bodies bind to receptors, enter cells, forming an intracellular reticulate body. Dividing reticulate bodies form new elementary bodies. Reticulate bodies form inclusion bodies in the host cell.
- *Chlamydia trachomatis*—Sensitive to sulfa drugs, stain with iodine (glycogen staining). Serotypes A, B, C cause trachoma, a chronic follicular keratoconjunctivitis, often resulting in blindness.
- Serotypes D–K cause reproductive tract infections, pneumonia, inclusion conjunctivitis. Chlamydial genital infections are widespread and common. Neonatal infections often result in inclusion conjunctivitis. Treat with erythromycins or tetracyclines.
- Serotypes L1, L2, and L3 cause lymphogranuloma venereum.
- Identify genital infections with molecular probes, fluorescent antibody (FA) staining for tissues, grow in McCoy cell cultures.
- *Chlamydia psittaci* uses birds as primary hosts. Humans develop an atypical pneumonia from inhaling the organism. Diagnosis is usually serology, not iodine staining.
- *Chlamydia pneumoniae* (TWAR)—human bronchitis, pneumonia, sinusitis. Treat with azithromycin.

Mycoplasma

Bacteria with no cell wall.

- Grown on laboratory media; do not Gram stain.
- *Mycoplasma pneumoniae*—causes sore throat through atypical pneumonia (walking pneumonia). Treat with tetracyclines or erythromycins.
- *U. urealyticum*—urethritis, prostatitis. Tiny colonies.
- Free radicals of oxygen (superoxides) kill anaerobic bacteria exposed to air. Superoxide dismutase is a potent bacterial antioxidant. The perixodases in bacteria are protective.
- Obligate anaerobes: Lack catalase and/or superoxide dismutase and susceptible to oxidative damage, foul smelling, produce gas in tissue (e.g., *Actinomyces*, *Bacteroides*, and *Clostridium*).
- Superoxide dismutase catalyzes: $2O_2^- + 2H^+ \rightarrow H_2O_2 + O_2$
- Catalase catalyzes: $2H_2O_2 \rightarrow 2H_2O + O_2$
- Myeloperoxidase catalyzes: $Cl^- + H_2O_2 \rightarrow ClO^- + H_2O$
- NADPH oxidase catalyzes: $NADPH + 2O_2 \rightarrow 2O_2^- + H^+ NADP^+$
- Sites of action of antimicrobial agents include cell-wall synthesis, cell-membrane integrity, DNA replication, protein synthesis, DNA-dependent RNA polymerase, folic acid metabolism.

MYCOLOGY

- Fungi (molds and yeasts) are eukaryotic—cell membranes have ergosterol (not cholesterol); target for imidazole, amphoteracin B, and nystatin antifungal.
- Fungal structures—hyphae (molds) or yeast.
  - Dimorphism—change from hyphae to yeast forms.
  - Hyphae grow into a mycelium; septate—cross-walls in hyphae; nonseptate—no cross-walls.
  - Yeasts—oval cells that replicate by budding.
  - Spores—reproductive devices—blastoconidia—yeast buds, conidia—hyphae, (macro- and microforms); endospores—*Coccidioides immitis*; arthroconidia—hyphae fragmentation.
- Laboratory—Sabouraud's agar-standard fungal medium.
  - Identity—based on morphology, biochemical test, immunologic tests, or genetic probes.
- Dermatophytes.
  - *Malassezia furfur*—hypopigmentation of skin.
  - *Trichophyton*—skin, hair, nails; *Microsporum*—hair and skin; *Epidermophyton*—nail and skin.
  - Tineas—ringworm (Tinea capitis—hair, Tinea corporis—skin, Tinea cruris—groin, Tinea pedis—foot).
  - *Candida*—pseudohyphae and yeast forms—normal flora—opportunist in immunocompromised patients.

- *Sporothrix schenckii*—dimorphic fungus—plants—transmission on thorns, etc., lymphotics involved.
- Thermally dimorphic fungi—systemic infections.
  - *Histoplasma capsulatum*—fungus in the environment with tuberculate macroconidia; small, oval budding yeast in cells of the RES.
  - Central U.S.—river valleys.
    - Primary disease—asymptomatic to pneumonia.
    - Systematic—especially in AIDS patients with mucocutaneous lesions common.
  - Laboratory—history plus blood smears and culture.
- *C. immitis*—environment (southwest U.S.—sandy)—hyphae develop into arthroconidia; inhaled arthroconidia develop into spherules (endospores).
  - Primary disease—(valley fever)—asymptomatic to self-limited pneumonia; disseminated form (certain HLA types, pregnancy, and immunocompromised)—to skin, bone, joints, and meninges).
  - Laboratory—culture (hazardous); sputum, urine, bronchial washes may show spherules.
- *Blastomyces dermatitidis*—environment—hyphae with conidia on stalks; tissue—large yeast with broad-based bud.
  - Same geographical area as *Histoplasma conidia* are inhaled.
  - Primary disease—pneumonia.
  - Laboratory—large yeast, broad-based buds.

Opportunistic Fungi
- *Aspergillus fumigatus*—hyphae with branches at acute angles and small conidia. Ubiquitous in environment. Fungus balls in lung cavities; invasive disease possible.
- *Candida albicans*—yeast and pseudohyphae normal mucocutaneous flora—oral thrush (infants and antibiotic users).
  - Endocarditis—IV drug abusers/indwelling catheters.
- *Cryptococcus neoformans*—yeast with large capsule.
  - Environment—soil with bird droppings.
  - Disease—pulmonary (often asymptomatic) in pigeon breeders; meningitis in AIDS patients and cancer patients.
  - Laboratory—latex agglutination—CSF (capsule antigen); india ink wet mount—capsules.
- *Mucor, Rhizopus, Absidia*—nonseptate hyphae.
  - Environment—common organisms.
  - Opportunists—rhinocerebral infections.
  - Laboratory—broad, nonseptate hyphae with 90° angles on branching.
- *Pneumocystis carinii*—exposure common—seldom disease except in immunocompromised (AIDS patients, etc.). Interstitial pneumonia presentation.
  - Laboratory—H and E tissue stains, silver stains.

PARASITOLOGY

- Protozoa are single-celled animals; trophozoites are motile, while cysts are involved in transmission.
- Amebas.
  - *Entamoeba histolytica*—disease of the large intestine; amebic dysentery—trophozoites feed on red blood cells (RBCs), causing ulcers. Also liver and lung abscesses possible.
  - *Naegleria*—free-living ameba in hot-water sources; primary amebic meningoencephalitis (PAM). Rapid onset of symptoms, with death possible in days.
  - Acanthamoeba—free-living amebas.
- Flagellates.
  - *Giardia lamblia*—worldwide distribution, animal reservoirs. Cysts in water sources; trophozoites attach to intestine, causing watery diarrhea and malabsorption. Cramping, light-colored, fatty stools. Also in day-care centers.
  - *Trichomonas vaginalis*—Trophozoite with undulating membrane and polar flagella. Presents with fishy-smelling, yellow discharge. Males usually asymptomatic, sexually transmitted.
  - *Trypanosoma*—flagellates, tsetse fly vector. African sleeping sickness.
  - *Trypanosoma cruzi*—Chagas' disease, kissing bug vector. South and Central America.
  - *Leishmania*—sandfly vectors. Visceral, cutaneous, and mucocutaneous lesions.
- Sporozoans—sexual and asexual life cycle forms.
  - *Cryptosporidium parvum*—U.S. waters, causes a self-limited diarrhea.
  - *Plasmodium* species cause malaria. *Anopheles* mosquito vectors. Complicated life cycles. *Plasmodium vivax, Plasmodium ovale, Plasmodium malariae, Plasmodium falciparum*.
  - *Toxoplasma gondii*—reservoir is cats. Humans ingest cysts from cat feces or undercooked meats. Special danger in human fetus development.
- Flukes.
  - *Fasciolopsis buski*—intestinal, cysts on water plants ingested, diarrhea.
  - *Clonorchis sinensis*—liver, from raw or undercooked fish. Biliary tree localization and liver location.
  - *Fasciola hepatica*—sheep liver fluke. Ingestion of metacercariae on aquatic plants.
  - *Schistosoma*—blood flukes.
- Cestodes—segmented flatworms with complicated life cycles.
  - *Taenia solium* (pork) and *Taenia saganata* (beef)—larval forms in undercooked meat. Adult tapeworms develop in the intestine.
  - *Diphyllobothrium latum*—fish tapeworm. Fish in freshwater lakes, undercooked fish ingested. Depletes host of vitamin B_{12}.
  - *Echinococcus granulosis*—tissue cestode. Humans are intermediate hosts and ingest eggs from sheepdog feces.

- Nematodes—roundworms.
  - *Ascaris lumbricoides*—may cause intestinal blockage.
  - *Enterobius vermicularis* (pinworm)—eggs in bedclothing, etc. Autoinoculation common. Widespread in U.S.
  - *Necator americanus*—New World hookworm.
  - *Ancylostoma duodenale*—Old World hookworm. Eggs in soil, penetrate bare feet.
  - *Strongyloides stercoralis* (threadworm)—tropics, southwest U.S., similar to hookworms.
  - *Trichuris trichiura* (whipworm)—tropics. Eggs ingested, poor sanitation. Causes mucoid or bloody diarrhea.
  - *Trichinella spiralis* (pork roundworm)—larvae ingested in pork or wild game meat. Larvae may calcify in muscle of intermediate host.
- Tissue nematodes—filarial worms. None are significant in U.S.
  - *Onchocerca volvulus*—river blindness, blackfly vector.
  - Loa loa—biting fly vector.
  - *Wuchereria bancrofti*—mosquito vectors. May cause elephantiasis.

IMMUNOLOGY

- Two types of immune response: (1) Adaptive or acquired (specific), (2) innate (native or nonadaptive).
- Innate immunity: Nonspecific, no immunological memory, first line of defense (epithelial), biochemical defenses (stomach $\downarrow$pH, GI proteolytic enzymes and bile), phagocytes (polymorphonuclear neutrophils [PMNs] and monocytes, macrophages), Soluble mediators (complement, acute-phase proteins such as C-reactive protein, cytokines such as ILs, IFNs, CSFs), inflammation (C5a: chemotaxis, C3b: opsonization, neutrophils).
- Adaptive immunity: Specific, antigen-driven, possesses discrimination and memory, divided into (1) humoral immunity (B cells, plasma cells) and (2) cell-mediated immunity (T helper, T cytotoxic).
- Antibodies (B lymphocytes/plasma cells): Main functions are (1) *neutralize* toxins/viruses, (2) *opsonize* bacteria, (3) *complement activation.*
- Antibodies (five isotypes): IgG, IgA, IgM, IgD, IgE (based on Fc heavy-chain differences), two light chains and two heavy chains held together by S-H bridges, hinge region is polyproline, paratope binds antigen and composed of heavy and light chain. Pepsin yields F(ab)$_2$, papain yields two "useless arms."
- Antibody concentrations (serum): IgG > IgA > IgM > IgD > IgE.
- IgG: Transplacental (Rh incompatibility, hemolytic disease of newborn), 80% of serum antibody, binds (activates) complement, four subclasses, main antibody in secondary response.
- IgA: Secretory antibody, serum (monomer), secretions (dimers), two subclasses, dimer (J chain), does not bind complement.

- IgM: Pentamer, binds complement, first to appear after infection, elevated in congenital/perinatal infections.
- IgD: Susceptible to proteolytic degradation, found with surface IgM on mature B lymphocytes.
- IgE: Cytotropic/reaginic antibody, allergy antibody, type I hypersensitivity (mast cells/basophils protective in worm infections), lowest concentration in serum.
- Bence Jones proteins: Multiple myeloma—large amounts of κ/λ light chains in urine excretion.
- Natural killer cells: Marker is CD16 (IgG Fc receptor).
- B cells: Antibody producers contributing to allergy (IgE), autoimmunity, host defense (opsonize, neutralize, complement activate).
- B cell markers: Fc receptor, C3 receptor, CD21 (receptor for EB virus), CD10 (CALLA).
- T cells: Host defense (fungi, viruses, *M. tuberculosis*), allergy (type IV), antibody regulation, graft/tumor rejection.
- T cell markers: CD2, TCRαβ-CD3, CD4 (HIV) or CD8, CD44 (migration).
- Complement deficiencies: (1) C1 esterase inhibitor: angioedema; (2) DAF: paroxysmal nocturnal hemoglubinuria; (3) C3: severe, recurrent infections (sinus and respiratory).
- Major histocompatibility complex (MHC) Class I: Exists on all nucleated cells.
- MHC Class II: Exists on antigen-presenting cells (macrophages/dendritic cells), important to organ rejection.
- Cytokines: IFN (antiviral), TNF (inflammation, fever, acute-phase reactants, cachexia), IL-1 (fever/pyrogen, acute-phase proteins), IL-2 (T cell stimulator), IL-3 (bone marrow stimulator), IL-4 (IgE production), IL-5 (proeosinophil, antihelminths), IL-6 (acute-phase proteins, B cell differentiation), IL-8 (inflammation, chemotaxis), IL-12 (NK cell stimulator, T_H1 stimulator, active cytotoxic lymphocyte stimulator, promotes cell-mediated immunity).
- Acute-phase cytokines: IL-1, IL-6, TNF-α.
- Mitogens: B lymphocytes (LPS), T lymphocytes (PHA and Con A), both B and T cells (PWM).
- ELISA presumptive diagnosis of HIV infection, western blot definitive diagnosis of HIV infection → both detecting anti-HIV antibodies in patient sera; detection of HIV RNA by nucleic acid amplification of viral load is best predictor of "progression to AIDS."
- Immunodeficiencies: (1) Primary—rare and *cause* disease; (2) secondary—common and the *result* of disease.
- Primary immunodeficiencies: Bruton's agammaglobulinemia—no B cells, low antibodies, small tonsils, only males; DiGeorge's syndrome (congenital thymic aplasia)—third and fourth pharyngeal pouches development failure, no thymus, no T cells, no parathyroid (hypocalcemia), and recurrent viral, fungal, protozoal infections; severe combined immunodeficiency disease (SCID)—no T or B cells,

defective IL-2 receptor, deficiency adenosine enzyme, recurrent infections (viral, bacterial, fungal, protozoal); Wiskott Aldrich—B and T cell deficiency, low IgM, high IgA, normal IgE; ataxia telangiectasia—defective DNA repair; Chédiak-Higashi disease—autosomal-recessive defect in phagocytosis; chronic granulomatous disease (CGD)—NADPH oxidase deficiency, increased opportunistic pathogens, phagocytic deficiency; chronic mucocutaneous candidiasis—*C. albicans* T cell dysfunction.

- Immunodeficiency characterized by unusual and recurrent infections:
  - B cell (antibody) deficiency—bacterial infections.
  - T cell deficiency—viral, fungal, and protozoal infections.
  - Phagocytic cells deficiency—pyogenic infections (bacterial), skin infections, systemic bacterial opportunistic infections.
  - Complement deficiencies—pyogenic infections (bacterial).
- Hypersensitivity: (1) Type I (anaphylaxis, immediate-type hypersensitivity); (2) type II (cytotoxic hypersensitivity); (3) type III (immune complex hypersensitivity); type IV (cell-mediated, delayed-type hypersensitivity).
- Type I: Mast cell/basophil, IgE, vasoactive amines, asthma, anaphylaxis, local wheal, and flare.
- Type II: IgM, IgG bind antigen and lyse cell, autoimmune hemolytic anemia, Goodpasture's syndrome, erythroblastosis fetalis.
- Type III: Immune complex, serum sickness, Arthus reaction → antibody-antigen complexes.
- Type IV: Lymphokines released from activated T lymphocytes, TB skin test, contact dermatitis, transplant rejection.
- Autoantibodies: Systemic lupus (antinuclear antibodies, anti-dsDNA, anti-Smith); drug-induced lupus (antihistone); rheumatoid arthritis (anti-IgG); celiac disease (antigliadin), Goodpasture's syndrome (antibasement membrane); Hashimoto's thyroiditis (antimicrosomal); scleroderma CREST (anticentromere); scleroderma diffuse (anti-scl-70).
- Active immunity: Induced after exposure to foreign antigens, memory established, slow onset.
- Vaccines: (1) Capsular polysaccharide vaccines (*Streptococcus, N. meningitidis, H. influenzae*); (2) toxoid vaccines (*C. diphtheriae, C. tetani, B. pertussis*); (3) purified protein vaccines (*B. pertussis, Borrelia burgdorferi, B. anthracis*); (4) live, attenuated bacterial vaccines (*Mycobacterium bovis* for tuberculosis/BCG, *F. tularensis*); (5) killed bacterial vaccines (*V. cholerae, Y. pestis, R. rickettsiae*/typhus, *C. burnetii*/Q fever); (6) killed, live, attenuated, and polysaccaride vaccines (*S. typhi*).
- Adjuvants (human vaccines): Aluminum hydroxide or lipid.
- Passive immunity: Administration of preformed antibody in immune globulin preparations, no memory established, rapid onset (e.g., tetanus antitoxin, botulinum antitoxin, diphtheria antitoxin), antitoxin = immune globulins.

Physiology and Molecular Microbiology

Questions

DIRECTIONS: Each question below contains four or more suggested responses. Select the **one best** response to each question.

1. Penicillinase isolated from *Staphylococcus aureus* inactivates 6-aminopenicillanic acid (shown below) by breaking which of the following numbered bonds?

a. 1
b. 2
c. 3
d. 4
e. 5

2. Which of the following bacterial transport methods is energy-independent?

a. ATP-dependent active transport
b. Facilitated diffusion
c. Group translocation
d. Proton gradient energized active transport
e. Simple diffusion

3. Iron is essential in bacterial metabolism. When bacteria invade the human host they must capture iron in order to survive. Which of the macromolecules listed below is important in bacterial iron metabolism?

a. Ferric oxide
b. Lactoferrin
c. Lipopolysaccharide (LPS)
d. Siderophores
e. Transferrin

4. An aliquot of *Escherichia coli* is treated with ethylenediaminetetraacetic acid (EDTA). The first wash is analyzed and found to contain alkaline phosphatase, DNase, and penicillinase. Which of the following is the anatomic area of the cell most likely affected by the EDTA?

a. Chromosome
b. Mesosomal space
c. Periplasmic space
d. Plasma membrane
e. Slime layer

Item 5–6

Oxygen is poison to some bacterial cells. These cells are termed *anaerobes.* Other bacteria, termed *aerobes* and *facultative anaerobes,* withstand oxygen toxicity; that is, they can grow in the presence of O_2. The following two equations are critical for bacteria.

1. $2O^{2-} + 2H^+ \rightarrow H_2O_2 + O_2$
2. $H_2O_2 + H_2A^* \rightarrow 2H_2O + A$

*"A" may be a number of chemical groups.

5. Reaction 1 is catalyzed by which of the following?

a. ATPase
b. Catalase
c. Oxygen permease
d. Peroxidase
e. Superoxide dismutase

6. Reaction 2 is catalyzed by which of the following?

a. ATPase
b. Flavoprotein oxidase
c. Oxygen permease
d. Peroxidase
e. Superoxide dismutase

7. A bacterium is examined and found to lack superoxide dismutase, catalase, and peroxidase. Which of the following statements best describes this bacterium?

a. This bacterium does not produce peroxide
b. This bacterium does not produce superoxide
c. This bacterium is an anaerobe
d. This bacterium is more virulent than one containing the three enzymes
e. This bacterium will survive in an O_2 environment

Item 8–9

A 20-year-old pregnant female patient presents to the emergency room with a four-day history of fever, chills, and myalgia. Two days prior to this she had noted painful genital lesions. Pelvic examination revealed extensive vesicular and ulcerative lesions on the left labia minora and majora with marked edema. The cervix had exophytic (outward-growing) necrotic ulcerations. Specimens were taken to test for *Neisseria gonorrhoeae, Treponema pallidum, Haemophilus ducreyi, Chlamydia trachomatis,* and herpes simplex virus type 2.

8. You decide to use newly purchased cutting-edge technology to rapidly identify the infecting pathogen. Real-time polymerase chain reaction requires which of the following reaction ingredient sets?

a. Specimen (template DNA), forward primer, reverse primer, polymerase (Taq), dNTPs, $MgCl_2$ hepes buffer, H_2O, and fluorescent reporter (i.e. SYBR, green I)
b. Specimen (template DNA), forward primer, reverse primer, polymerase (Taq), dNTPs, $MgCl_2$, hepes buffer, and H_2O
c. Specimen (template DNA), forward primer only, polymerase (Taq), dNTPs, $MgCl_2$, hepes buffer, and H_2O
d. Specimen (template DNA), reverse primer only, polymerase (Taq), dNTPs, $MgCl_2$, hepes buffer, and H_2O
e. Specimen (template DNA), forward primer, reverse primer, dNTPs, $MgCl_2$, hepes buffer, H_2O, and fluorescent reporter (i.e. SYBR-green I)

9. Real-time SYBR-green PCR reveals the following results:

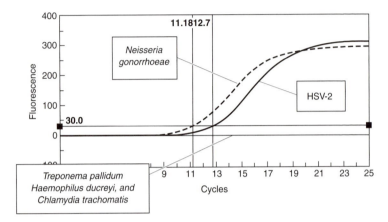

Which of the following is true?

a. The woman is infected with N. gonorrhoeae, T. pallidum, H. ducreyi, C. trachomatis, and herpes simplex virus type 2
b. The woman is infected with only herpes simplex type 2
c. The woman is infected with only N. gonorrhoeae
d. The woman is infected with both N. gonorrhoeae and herpes simplex type 2
e. The woman is not infected with any of the abovementioned pathogens

10. Reversion of N. gonorrhoeae from a fimbriated (fim 1) to a nonfimbriated (fim 2) state would result in which one of the following phenomena?

a. A negative capsule strain
b. Death of the organism
c. Inability of N. gonorrhoeae to colonize the mucosal epithelium
d. Loss of serologic specificity
e. Reversion to a gram-positive stain

11. An unknown isolate is recognized serologically as *Salmonella enteritidis* serovar *newport*. A mutant of this organism has lost region 1 (O-specific polysaccharide) of its lipopolysaccharide. This mutant would be identified as which of the following?

a. *Arizona*
b. *Salmonella typhi*
c. *Salmonella newport*
d. *S. enteritidis*
e. *S. enteritidis* serovar *newport*

12. Certain enzymes catalyze the cross-linking of peptidoglycan, a unique constituent of bacterial cell walls. Which of the following may be a factor in antibiotic resistance, the target of which is cell-wall synthesis?

a. Bactoprenol
b. DNA gyrase
c. Penicillin-binding proteins (PBPs)
d. Reverse transcriptase
e. RNA polymerase

13. Selective inhibition of synthesis of dipicolinic acid (structure shown below) would most likely inhibit the formation of which of the following structures?

a. Bacterial flagella
b. Bacterial spores
c. Eukaryotic cilia
d. Eukaryotic flagella
e. Fimbriae

Item 14–16

Following is the growth curve of *E. coli* growing in a nutrient medium at 35°C with both O_2 and added CO_2 present.

Growth curve—*E. Coli*

The following descriptions are given for the phases of this bacterial growth curve:

A. Lag phase
B. Log phase
C. Stationary phase
D. Death phase

14. In which of the phases would growth not be detectable?

a. Lag phase
b. Log phase
c. Stationary phase
d. Death phase

15. Treatment of the culture with gentamicin, an inhibitor of protein synthesis, would have maximal effect on which of the phases?

a. Lag phase
b. Log phase
c. Stationary phase
d. Death phase

16. If logarithmic growth could be sustained for 48 hours the mass of bacterial cells would equal a volume 500 times that of the planet Earth. Which of the following are limiting factors in microbial growth?

a. Accumulation of oxygen-free radicals
b. Accumulation of peroxide
c. Accumulation of toxic products in the growth medium
d. Loss of superoxide dismutase
e. Oxygen

17. Ideally, an antibiotic should focus on a microbial target not found in mammalian cells. By this standard, which of the following antibiotic agents would be expected to be most toxic to humans?

a. Bacitracin
b. Cephalosporin
c. Mitomycin
d. Penicillin
e. Vancomycin

Item 18–19

18. After obtaining spinal fluid from a patient presenting with meningitis, a Gram stain is performed. Which of the following is the correct order of procedural steps when performing the Gram stain?

a. Fixation, crystal violet, alcohol/acetone decolorization, safranin
b. Fixation, crystal violet, iodine treatment, alcohol/acetone decolorization, safranin
c. Fixation, crystal violet, iodine treatment, safranin
d. Fixation, crystal violet, safranin
e. Fixation, safranin, iodine treatment, alcohol/acetone decolorization, crystal violet

19. While performing the Gram stain you mistakenly forget the iodine treatment step. Which of the following is correct?

a. All the cells will be blue
b. All the cells will be decolorized
c. All the cells will be purple
d. All the cells will be red
e. All the cells will lyse, thus no Gram stain results will be obtained
f. Half of the cells will be red and the other half will be blue

20. *E. coli* has two major porins located in the outer membrane. Which of the following is the function of porins?

a. Diffusion of safranin from the cell, thereby rendering the cell gram-negative
b. Metabolism of phosphorylated intermediates
c. Serologic stabilization of the O antigen
d. Stabilization of the mesosome
e. Transfer of small molecules through the outer membrane

21. A 21-year-old man was bitten by a tick in Oregon. Two years later, during the course of routine screening for an unknown ailment, a screening Lyme disease test was performed, which was negative. A western blot strip (IgG) showed the following pattern:

Gp66

Which of the following is the correct interpretation of the test?

a. The patient has acute Lyme disease
b. The patient has chronic Lyme disease
c. The patient should be tested for HIV on the basis of the western blot
d. The pattern may represent nonspecific reactivity
e. The screening test should be repeated

22. Early attempts at the polymerase chain reaction (PCR) used *E. coli* DNA polymerase. This was replaced with DNA polymerase from *Thermus aquaticus* ("Taq" polymerase). Which of the following is the primary advantage in using this enzyme?

a. It is cheaper than *E. coli* polymerase
b. Specificity is increased because nonspecific hybridization of primers does not occur
c. Use of Taq polymerase enables lower temperatures to be used
d. Use of Taq polymerase results in fewer PCR cycles
e. Upon repeated cycling, Taq polymerase becomes denatured, which causes less interference with the hybridization process

Item 23–25

You have been asked to design a nucleic acid amplification test for a rarely isolated bacterium. There are several questions that you must ask in order to develop a test that could be used to diagnose disease.

23. Assume, initially, that the polymerase chain reaction (PCR) will amplify any DNA, human or microbial. Which of the following is the best way to prevent contamination of the PCR process?

a. Do all of the work under a hood
b. Incorporate self-sterilizing agents into the PCR mixture
c. Use universal precautions
d. Wash benches with bleach
e. Wear gloves

24. You must choose primers for this PCR. *Primers* are small pieces of nucleic acid that recognize a pair of unique sites on the bacterial chromosome. For an optimum test to be developed, which of the following characteristics is the least desirable?

a. Ability to be constructed by a synthesizer
b. Ability to serve as a template for replication
c. Complementary to sequences on the bacterial chromosome
d. That the sequences are widely recognized by many bacterial species
e. Uniqueness to the organism that you wish to detect

25. You have chosen the primers for the PCR that you have designed. You have also developed a reaction mixture that contains, among other substances, a polymerase enzyme. After the primer pairs have been amplified, they must be detected. Which of the following detection methods is most sensitive (that is, will detect the highest number of amplicons)?

a. Capture of the amplicons on a solid phase followed by an enzyme immunoassay
b. Ethidium staining of the amplified products (amplicons)
c. Labeling of the amplicons with fluorescent dyes
d. Microscopy
e. Southern blot

26. Which one of the following statements about the *E. coli* cells shown in the photomicrograph below is true?

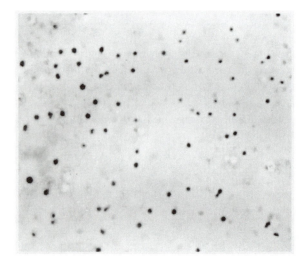

a. They are commonly referred to as endospores
b. They are osmotically stable
c. They can result from treatment with penicillin
d. They have formed cell walls but have become coccoid
e. Treatment of the parent *E. coli* with lysozyme has no effect

27. The purpose of gene cloning is to produce large amounts of genes in pure form. The sequence of the cloning process is critical to the production of clones. Which of the following steps initializes the cloning process?

a. Amplification of source DNA
b. Detection and purification of clones
c. Incorporation of a cloning vector into the host cell
d. Isolation and fragmentation of source DNA
e. Joining of host DNA to a cloning vector

28. Nucleic acid probes are useful not only for searching for genes in the cloning host but also for searching for genes or gene fragments in patient specimens. Which one of the following statements is true of nucleic acid probes?

a. Nucleic acid probes are not as sensitive as traditional culture methods for detection of pathogenic microorganisms
b. Only DNA can be used as a probe
c. Primers are labeled to allow detection, but probes are unlabeled
d. Probes can be designed so that they can detect very specific pieces of a nucleic acid, for example, a penicillin-resistant gene
e. Probes may contain any part of the base sequence of the gene of interest

29. DNA from a host sample can be amplified by the polymerase chain reaction. Which of the following is required for PCR?

a. A heat-sensitive DNA polymerase enzyme
b. A single nucleotide primer
c. An ultracentrifuge
d. A universal probe to detect the amplified product
e. Knowledge of the genetic sequence to be amplified

Item 30–33

The following five growth curves are lettered (A–E) corresponding to an expected growth curve if certain antibiotics were added to an exponentially growing culture of E. coli. The arrow indicates when antibiotics were added to the growing culture.

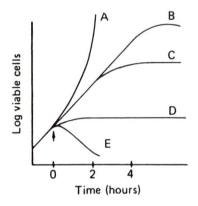

30. Chloramphenicol treatment would be expected to produce which one of the following growth curves?

a. A
b. B
c. C
d. D
e. E

31. Penicillin would be expected to produce which one of the following growth curves?

a. A
b. B
c. C
d. D
e. E

32. Sulfonamide would be expected to produce which one of the following growth curves?

a. A
b. B
c. C
d. D
e. E

33. If no antibiotics were added to the exponentially growing culture, which one of the following growth curves would result?

a. A
b. B
c. C
d. D
e. E

Item 34–36

DNA can be transferred from one bacterium to another by a number of processes.

34. Uptake by a recipient cell of soluble DNA released from a donor cell is defined as which one of the following?

a. Competence
b. Conjugation
c. Recombination
d. Transduction
e. Transformation

35. Transfer of a donor chromosome fragment by a temperate bacterial virus is defined as which one of the following?

a. Competence
b. Conjugation
c. Recombination
d. Transduction
e. Transformation

36. Direct transfer of a plasmid between two bacteria is defined as which one of the following?

a. Competence
b. Conjugation
c. Recombination
d. Transduction
e. Transformation

37. After incubating a culture of five *E. coli* bacteria for two hours, the following graph was constructed. Which of the following represents the number of *E. coli* now present in this culture?

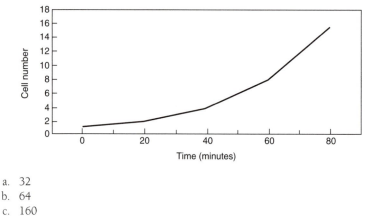

a. 32
b. 64
c. 160
d. 320
e. 640

38. Which of the following is true of Koch's postulates?

a. The causal organism must be isolated, grown in pure culture, cause disease in a healthy susceptible animal, and ultimately be recovered from the inoculated animal
b. The causal organism must be isolated, grown in pure culture, cause disease in a previously immunized (to the causal organism) animal, and ultimately be recovered from the inoculated animal
c. The causal organism need only be isolated and grown in pure culture
d. The causal organism may be inferred through an extensive history and physical of the diseased animal
e. The causal organism must cause repeated symptoms (illness) in the same (original) animal

39. The following diagram illustrates the cell wall of gram-negative bacteria.

Which of the following statements is indicative of the contents of the indicated (arrow) portion in the preceding diagram?

a. Genetic material such as DNA or RNA
b. Hydrolytic enzymes such as β-lactamases
c. Lipid A
d. Lipopolysaccharide (LPS)
e. Teichoic acid

40. In comparing viruses with prions, which of the following is true?

a. Both prions and viruses contain some form and quantity of nucleic acid, either DNA, RNA, or both
b. Both viruses and prions upon infection induce an antibody response in the host
c. Both viruses and prions upon infection induce an inflammatory response in the host
d. Conventional viruses are rapidly inactivated by ultraviolet light or heat, whereas prions are not
e. Both viral and prion proteins are encoded by viral genes

Item 41–42

Mutations are heritable changes in the structure of genes.

41. The replacement mutation of a purine by a pyrimidine or vice versa is known as which one of the following?

a. Inversion
b. Missense
c. Nonsense
d. Transition
e. Transversion

42. The replacement mutation in a codon changing the mRNA transcript to a different amino acid is known as which one of the following?

a. Inversion
b. Missense
c. Nonsense
d. Transition
e. Transversion

Item 43–47

43. A patient presents to the emergency room with vomiting, diarrhea, high fever, and delirium. Upon physical exam, you notice large, painful buboes and disseminated intravascular coagulation. Laboratory diagnosis of aspirate taken from the bubo reveals bipolar staining resembling a safety pin. As part of your treatment, you immediately give which of the following?

a. Ceftazidine
b. Ceftriaxone
c. Penicillin
d. Streptomycin
e. Vancomycin

44. Which of the following is a preferred third-generation cephalosporin with good activity against childhood meningitis?

a. Ceftazidine
b. Ceftriaxone
c. Penicillin
d. Streptomycin
e. Vancomycin

45. A patient presents to the emergency room with a progressive fever, cough, and general malaise. History determines that he works with sheep on a farm and had just been involved in wool harvesting. You immediately begin treatment with which of the following?

a. Ceftazidine
b. Ceftriaxone
c. Penicillin
d. Streptomycin
e. Vancomycin

46. Which of the following is a third-generation cephalosporin with primary activity against *Pseudomonas aeruginosas*?

a. Ceftazidine
b. Ceftriaxone
c. Penicillin
d. Streptomycin
e. Vancomycin

47. Laboratory results of a clinical specimen from a patient with hospital-acquired pneumonia reveal the presence of *S. aureus* with a methicillin-resistant plasmid. You immediately begin treatment with which of the following?

a. Ceftazidine
b. Ceftriaxone
c. Penicillin
d. Streptomycin
e. Vancomycin

48. Which one of the following antibiotics inhibits dihydrofolate reductase?

a. Amdinocillin
b. Amphotericin
c. Chloramphenicol
d. Penicillin
e. Trimethoprim

49. Which one of the following antibiotics binds to penicillin-binding protein-2 (PBP-2)?

a. Amdinocillin
b. Amphotericin
c. Chloramphenicol
d. Penicillin
e. Trimethoprim

50. Which one of the following antibiotics inhibits the final peptide bond between d-alanine and glycine?

a. Amdinocillin
b. Amphotericin
c. Chloramphenicol
d. Penicillin
e. Trimethoprim

51. Which one of the following antibiotics binds sterols and alters membrane permeability?

a. Amdinocillin
b. Amphotericin
c. Chloramphenicol
d. Penicillin
e. Trimethoprim

52. Which one of the following antibiotics attaches to 50S ribosome and inhibits peptidyl transferase?

a. Amdinocillin
b. Amphotericin
c. Chloramphenicol
d. Penicillin
e. Trimethoprim

Item 53–57

The following diagram illustrates the amplification of DNA by PCR. There are at least four points in the PCR process (A–D) that are critical to the reaction.

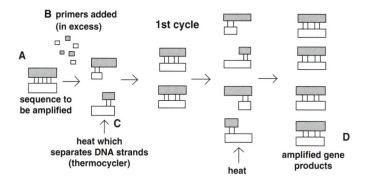

53. The Southern blot detection system for amplified PCR products fails to function. Which one of the following would be affected?

a. A
b. B
c. C
d. D

54. DNA does not hybridize with the primers. Which one of the following would be affected?

a. A
b. B
c. C
d. D

55. The laboratory observes a series of false-positive results. Which one of the following processes would you suspect to be faulty?

a. A
b. B
c. C
d. D

56. The DNA strands fail to reanneal. Which one of the following processes would you suspect to be faulty?

a. A
b. B
c. C
d. D

57. The laboratory observes a series of false-negative results. Which one of the following processes would you suspect to be faulty?

a. A
b. B
c. C
d. D

Item 58–63

Bacteria or their components may be characterized by unique constituents or structures.

58. *Neisseria meningitidis*, group B, is characterized by which one of the following?

a. γ-glutamyl polypeptide
b. Hyaluronic acid
c. Outer-membrane proteins
d. Repeating polysaccharide capsule of glucose and glucuronic acid
e. Sialic acid polymers

59. Group A streptococci are characterized by which one of the following?

a. γ-glutamyl polypeptide
b. Hyaluronic acid
c. Outer-membrane proteins
d. Repeating polysaccharide capsule of glucose and glucuronic acid
e. Sialic acid polymers

60. Bacterial lipopolysaccharide (LPS) is characterized by which one of the following?

a. Glycolipids (waxes)
b. Ketodeoxyoctulonate (KDO)
c. Phospholipid
d. Repeating polysaccharide capsule of glucose and glucuronic acid
e. Ribitol teichoic acid

61. *Mycobacterium* cell walls are characterized by which one of the following?

a. Glycolipids (waxes)
b. Ketodeoxyoctulonate (KDO)
c. Phospholipid
d. Repeating polysaccharide capsule of glucose and glucuronic acid
e. Ribitol teichoic acid

62. *Bacillus anthracis* capsules consist of which one of the following?

a. γ-glutamyl polypeptide
b. Hyaluronic acid
c. Outer-membrane proteins
d. Repeating polysaccharide capsule of glucose and glucuronic acid
e. Sialic acid polymers

63. *Streptococcus pneumoniae* are characterized by which one of the following?

a. γ-glutamyl polypeptide
b. Hyaluronic acid
c. Outer-membrane proteins
d. Repeating polysaccharide capsule of glucose and glucuronic acid
e. Sialic acid polymers

Physiology and Molecular Microbiology

Answers

1. The answer is d. (*Levinson, pp 59–62. Ryan, pp 196–198.*) The structural integrity of the β-lactam ring in penicillins is essential for their antimicrobial activity. Many resistant strains of staphylococci produce an enzyme, penicillinase, that cleaves the β-lactam ring at the carbon-nitrogen bond. Other organisms, including certain coliform bacteria, produce an amidase enzyme that inactivates penicillin by disrupting the bond between the radical and nitrogen in the free amino group (1 in the diagram).

2. The answer is e. (*Ryan, pp 28–29.*) Almost no important nutrients enter the bacterial cell through simple diffusion, an exception being carbon dioxide and oxygen. Some diffusion, however, is facilitated by specific protein carriers. Most transport, except simple diffusion, is energy-dependent, particularly in gram-negative bacteria. Group translocation occurs in the absence of oxygen. For example, a simple carbohydrate such as glucose is phosphorylated enzymatically and is then transported into the cell.

3. The answer is d. (*Ryan, p 29.*) Siderophores such as aerobactin and enterobactin are chelators that trap iron Fe^{3+}. This Fe-chelator complex is actually transported inside the cell. Transferrin and lactoferrin are iron-binding proteins found in blood and milk. Ferric or iron oxide is rust, and lipopolysaccharide (LPS) is a microbial cell-wall constituent.

4. The answer is c. (*Levinson, p 6. Ryan, p 19.*) The periplasm is the space between the outer membrane and the plasma membrane of bacteria. The periplasmic space in *E. coli* has been shown to contain a number of proteins, sugars, amino acids, and inorganic ions. Ethylenediaminetetraacetic acid (EDTA) is a chelating agent that disrupts the cell walls of gram-negative bacteria.

5–6. The answers are 5-e, 6-d. (*Levinson, pp 14–15, 48. Ryan, p 31.*) Oxygen, when it is metabolized, gives rise to hydrogen peroxide (H_2O_2) and superoxide-anion (O_2). Both of these by-products are extremely toxic to cells. Peroxide is produced by many bacteria, particularly facultative anaerobes that use flavoprotein intermediates. H_2O_2 is degraded by peroxidases, as illustrated in equation 2. Superoxide is detoxified by a critical enzyme known as *superoxide dismutase*. Such metabolism also results in H_2O_2 production (equation 1). *Peroxidase* and *catalase* are often used interchangeably to describe H_2O_2 reactions. However, in equation 2 when the H_2A reactant is another H_2O_2 molecule, the enzyme is known as *catalase*. If H_2A is another intermediate, then the enzyme is known as *peroxidase*.

7. The answer is c. *(Levinson, pp 14–15, 88–89. Ryan, p 31.)* Superoxide dismutase is an enzyme found in both prokaryotic and eukaryotic cells that can survive in an environment of O_2. Lack of this enzyme, as well as peroxidase and catalase, ensures that a bacterium will not grow in the presence of O_2. Absence of these enzymes is not related to virulence, although ability to survive in an O_2-rich atmosphere may impart certain benefits to the proliferation of bacteria in the human host.

8–9. The answers are 8-a, 9-d. *(Ryan, pp 251–255.)* Although traditional PCR had many advantages in speeding up the process of detecting the presence/absence of DNA/RNA in a sample, it had many limitations, with end-point detection being its largest problem. End-point detection involves the need for running agarose gel electrophoresis of the PCR product to visualize the presence/absence of DNA/RNA in a sample. This is time consuming, messy, and, overall, not ideal in the clinical setting. This led to the development of an enhanced modality known as *real-time PCR*.

With the advent of real-time PCR, many of the limitations of traditional PCR have been overcome. Real-time PCR allows for the detection of PCR amplification during the early phases of the PCR reaction and therefore avoids the need for gel electrophoresis, thus minimizing time to detection. The same stage cycling (denaturation, annealing, extension) used in traditional PCR is also utilized in the real-time PCR system. The difference, however, exists in the dependence of real-time PCR on a fluorescent reporter for the detection and quantitation of target DNA. This reporter signal increases in direct proportion to the amount of PCR product (amplicon) in a reaction. By recording the amount of fluorescence emission at each cycle, it is possible to monitor the PCR reaction during the exponential phase where the first significant increase in the amount of PCR product correlates to the initial amount of target template. There are two general methods for the quantitative detection of the amplicon: (1) fluorescent probes (FAM, TAMRA, TET, ROX, etc.) or (2) DNA-binding agents (SYBR-green I, ethidium bromide, etc.).

SYBR-green is a dye that binds the minor groove of double-stranded DNA (dsDNA). When SYBR-green binds to dsDNA, the intensity of the fluorescent emissions increases. As more dsDNA amplicons are produced, the SYBR-green signal will increase, allowing for real-time analysis while the PCR reaction is running.

Real-time PCR is a powerful improvement over the traditional PCR system and can be applied to such investigations as (1) viral quantitation, (2) quantitation of gene expression, (3) array verification, (4) drug therapy efficacy, (5) DNA damage measurement, (6) quality control and assay validation, (7) pathogen detection (rapid and accurate), and (8) genotyping. A real-time PCR reaction, in addition to requiring the same ingredients as a regular PCR reaction (i.e., specimen/template DNA, forward primer, reverse primer, polymerase [Taq], dNTPs, $MgCl_2$, hepes buffer, H_2O), also requires the presence of a fluorescent reporter such as SYBR-green I. The diagram represented in question 9 was obtained using a Smart Cycler II® real-time PCR machine purchased from Cepheid®. Sigmoidal-shape curves indicate amplification in vitro and, hence, presence of *N. gonorrhoeae* and HSV-2 in the collected clinical sample. Horizontal lines represent no amplification and the absence of *T. pallidum, H. ducreyi,* and *C. trachomatis* in the obtained clinical sample. Real-time PCR is becoming inceasingly important in the clinical setting for rapid and sensitive identification of pathogens from clinically obtained samples, and thus should be a familiar process to every health care professional.

10. The answer is c. (*Levinson, pp 6, 12. Ryan, p 22.*) Bacteria may shift rapidly between the fimbriated (fim +) and the nonfimbriated (fim −) states. Fimbriae function as adhesions to specific surfaces and consequently play a major role in pathogenesis. Lack of fimbriae prevents colonization of the mucosal surface by the bacterium.

11. The answer is d. (*Levinson, pp 121–124. Ryan, pp 353, 362–363.*) Region 1 (the O-antigenic side chain of lipopolysaccharide) is responsible for the many serotypes of *Salmonella*. A mutant of *Salmonella* deficient in region 1 is not identified as a "newport," at least by virtue of its somatic antigen; biochemical identification of this mutant would be *S. enteritidis*. Loss of region 1 does not affect genus and species classification of *Salmonella*. Recently, however, it has been recommended that *Salmonella* be referred to by genus and serovar, that is, *Salmonella newport* or *Salmonella* serovar *newport*.

12. The answer is c. *(Levinson, pp 59–60, 73, 75–76. Ryan, pp 36, 196.)* Transpeptidases or penicillin-binding proteins (PBPs) combine with penicillin to keep the final cross-linking step in the synthesis of peptidoglycan in the cell wall. All of the other choices are involved in polymerization processes. Examples of polymerization include the cell membrane (bactoprenol) and synthesis of DNA and RNA.

13. The answer is b. *(Levinson, pp 6, 12–13. Ryan, pp 24–25.)* Dipicolinic acid, formed in the synthesis of diaminopimelate (DAP), is a prominent component of bacterial spores but is not found in vegetative cells or eukaryotic appendages or fimbrial structures. The calcium salt of dipicolinic acid apparently plays an important role in stabilizing spore proteins, but its mechanism of action is unknown. Dipicolinic acid synthetase is an enzyme unique to bacterial spores.

14–16. The answers are 14-a, 15-b, 16-c. *(Levinson, p 14. Ryan, pp 41–42.)* Bacterial growth curves are multiphasic. The lag phase is characterized by lack of growth but not necessarily metabolic activity. The bacteria are "adjusting" to their new environment. Depending on the bacteria, the temperature, nutrients, and pH, the microorganisms start dividing after a few hours and grow logarithmically for 12 to 18 hours. Toxins accumulate in the medium and nutrients become limiting. Oxygen and CO_2 are usually not limiting, as the gases freely diffuse into the growing culture. When death and growth of cells are equal, the stationary phase occurs. The death phase is characterized by a death rate that is more rapid than the growth rate. An antibiotic that inhibits protein synthesis would be optimally active in a rapidly dividing culture where proteins are being rapidly synthesized, that is, the logarithmic phase. Bacteria introduced into the human host may undergo similar phases of growth. However, other factors such as host defenses play a major role in limiting logarithmic growth, as does accumulation of toxic by-products as might occur in a closed-space infection such as an abscess.

17. The answer is c. (*Levinson, pp 59–60. Ryan, pp 215–216.*) Ideally, antibiotics should attack a microbial structure or function not found in human cells. Except for mitomycin, all the antibiotics listed in the question interfere with cell-wall synthesis in bacteria. Mitomycin inhibits DNA synthesis in both mammalian and microbial systems; viral DNA synthesis, however, is relatively resistant to mitomycin.

18–19. The answers are 18-b, 19-d. (*Levinson, pp 8, 53–57, 87–88. Ryan, pp 16, 232–233.*) First described in 1884 by a Danish physician, Hans Christian Gram, the Gram stain has proved to be one of the most useful diagnostic laboratory procedures in microbiology and medicine. The Gram stain procedure is characterized by the following steps: (1) *fixation* of the bacteria to the slide, (2) crystal violet (acridine dye) treatment, (3) iodine treatment, (4) *decolorization* using alcohol/acetone wash, and (4) *counterstaining* using safranin. Gram-positive bacteria have thick outer walls with no lipids, whereas gram-negative bacteria have a thin wall and an outer membrane. The difference between gram-positive and gram-negative organisms is in the cell-wall permeability to these complexes on treatment with mixtures of acetone and alcohol solvents. Thus, gram-positive bacteria retain purple iodine-dye complexes, whereas gram-negative bacteria do not retain these complexes when decolorized using an alcohol/acetone wash. If the iodine treatment step is omitted during the Gram stain process, the purple iodine-dye complexes will not form. The crystal violet will wash away during the alcohol/acetone decolorization washing step and all cells will appear *red*. Gram staining of pus or fluids along with clinical findings can guide the management of an infection before culture results are available in the clinical setting.

20. The answer is e. (*Levinson, p 6. Ryan, pp 19, 21.*) E. coli has two major porins, OMP C and OMP E (OMP is outer-membrane protein). A porin is a protein trimer with each subunit containing a pore with a diameter of 1 nm. Porins function in outer-membrane (OM) permeability. While porins are known to permit the transfer of small molecules across the OM, specific porins may also influence the diffusion of layer molecules. Also, porins can allow the passage of many antimicrobial drugs such as penicillin. Depending on charge, porins may also repel certain molecules, such as bile salts found in the intestinal environment.

21. The answer is d. (*Levinson, pp 155–157. Ryan, pp 434–437.*) The serologic diagnosis of Lyme disease is fraught with difficulty. Enzyme immunoassay (EIA) may be insensitive in the early stages of disease and may lack specificity in advanced stages. Western blot analysis of the antibody is the confirmatory test for Lyme disease, but it, too, is not 100% sensitive and specific. The western blot test detects antibodies to proteins and glycoproteins of *Borrelia burgdorferi*. Not all of these proteins are specific for the organism. For example, antibodies to Gp66 may reflect a cross-reaction, as many gram-negative bacteria have similar glycoproteins. For this reason, a western blot showing only antibodies to Gp66 is thought to be a nonspecific immune response.

22. The answer is b. (*Ryan, pp 251–253.*) DNA polymerase isolated from the hot springs thermophilic bacterium named *T. aquaticus* is essential for the PCR process because of its stability at high temperatures (95°C). While the *E. coli* enzyme can be used, the enzyme itself becomes denatured, fewer cycles are possible, and nonspecific reactions occur because of hybridization of primers to nontarget DNA. The use of Taq polymerase allows DNA copying at 72°C rather than 37°C, which further reduces nonspecific hybridization.

23–25. The answers are 23-b, 24-d, 25-e. (*Ryan, pp 251–255.*) The PCR has revolutionized the detection of infectious microorganisms, particularly those that are difficult to grow. During their normal practice, physicians will usually not be required to design a PCR test, but they should know some of the design elements of PCR so that they might better understand the results from these widely used tests.

One of the major problems of PCR in the past was contamination from extraneous nucleic acid. There are several ways to prevent contamination and the resulting falsely positive results. They include the use of separate laboratories, hoods, gloves, and surface disinfectants. The most effective method, however, is the use of internal sterilizing agents such as uracil N-glycosyls (UNG). These agents cross-link extraneous DNA so that the product cannot be amplified. Primers can now be purchased from a catalog and their sequence obtained online. Primers are easily synthesized, must be complementary to sequences on the bacterial chromosome, and when coupled to such sequences must promote replication. The specificity of PCR is a function of choosing a primer pair that is unique to the organism that you wish to detect. The PCR process is best explained by the "needle in the haystack" analogy. One needle in a haystack is difficult to find. However, if one needle becomes a million needles, then detection is easy. The same is true for nucleic acids. The amplicons (amplified nucleic acids) can be detected by a number of methods because they are so plentiful. These methods include specific staining with ethidium bromide of a gel containing these amplicons, and Southern blotting of the amplicons "tags" them so that they can be seen on photographic film. Amplicons are also bound to solid phases and detected with labeled enzymes or an instrument that reads a fluorescent tag. Microscopy is not used.

26. The answer is c. (*Levinson, p 8. Ryan, p 19.*) The organisms illustrated in the question are spheroplasts of *E. coli*. Lysozyme clears the b-1-4-glycosidic bond between *N*-acetylmuramic acid and *N*-acetylglucosamine. Spheroplasts are bacteria with cell walls that have been partially removed by the action of lysozyme or penicillin. Ordinarily, with disintegration of the walls, the cells undergo lysis; however, in a hypertonic medium, the cells persist and assume a spherical configuration. Endospores are formed by gram-positive bacteria in the genera *Bacillus* and *Clostridium*. It has also been shown that for *E. coli* and other gram-negative rods, exposure to minimal concentrations of antibiotics does not rupture the cell wall but promotes elongation of the cell by inhibiting the division cycle.

27. The answer is d. (*Ryan, pp 252–253.*) Gene cloning is a basic step in virtually every genetic engineering process. First, the source DNA is isolated and cut into small pieces and then attached to a cloning vector with DNA ligase. The cloning vectors are inserted into the host organism (usually a bacterium), and then the cloned DNA is isolated, identified, and purified. Amplification of source DNA is not a necessary step.

28. The answer is d. (*Ryan, pp 251–255.*) Nucleic acid probes, either DNA or RNA, are commonly used in clinical and research microbiology laboratories. These complementary pieces of nucleic acid bind to genes or gene parts of interest and are detected by their label, which may be either radioactive or nonradioactive. Probes, in general, are more sensitive than traditional growth-dependent methods, particularly for those microorganisms that either cannot be cultured or grow very slowly.

29. The answer is e. *(Ryan, pp 251–255.)* PCR is a widely used tool for amplification of small pieces of nucleic acid present in minute quantities. Once the sequence to be amplified is known, a specific forward and reverse primer is added. The temperature is alternately raised and lowered up to 45 to 50 times in the presence of a heat-resistant DNA polymerase from *T. aquaticus.* The amplified gene product is then detected by one of a number of techniques such as cloning, direct hybridization, agarose gel electrophoresis, and southern hybridization.

30–33. The answers are 30-d, 31-e, 32-c, 33-b. *(Levinson, pp 14, 59–60, 64, 66–68. Ryan, pp 35, 41–42, 194–199, 201–202, 204.)* Penicillin causes lysis of growing bacterial cells. Its antimicrobial effect stems from impairment of cell-wall synthesis. Because penicillin is bactericidal, the number of viable cells should fall immediately after introduction of the drug into the medium.

Both chloramphenicol and sulfonamides are bacteriostatic—that is, they retard cell growth without causing cell death. Chloramphenicol causes an immediate, reversible, bacteriostatic inhibition of protein synthesis. Sulfonamides, on the other hand, compete with para-aminobenzoic acid in the synthesis of folate; intracellular stores of folate are depleted gradually as the cells continue to grow.

The number of viable cells in a culture eventually will level off, even if no antibiotic is added to the environment. A key factor in this phenomenon is the limited availability of substrate.

34–36. The answers are 34-e, 35-d, 36-b. *(Levinson, pp 17–20. Ryan, pp 57–64.)* Transformation, transduction, and conjugation are critical processes in which DNA is transferred from one bacterium to another. Transformation, the passage of high-molecular-weight DNA from one bacterium to another, was first observed in pneumococci. Later studies have shown that, at least in *S. pneumoniae,* double-stranded DNA is "nicked" by a membrane-bound endonuclease, initiating DNA entry into the host cell. One of the nicked DNA strands is digested, and the other is integrated into the host genome. Transduction, which can affect many bacteria, is a process in which a fragment of donor chromosome is carried to a recipient cell by a temperate virus (bacteriophage). In generalized transduction, the phage virus can carry any segment of the donor chromosome; in restricted transduction, the phage carries only those chromosomal segments immediately adjacent to the site of prophage attachment. In conjugation, too, DNA is passed from one bacterium to another. However, instead of the transfer of soluble DNA, a small loop of DNA, called a *plasmid,* is passed between cells. Examples of plasmids are the sex factors and the resistance (R) factors.

37. The answer is d. (*Levinson, p 14.*) Bacteria reproduce by binary fission and thus undergo exponential (logarithmic) growth. In this question, the chart indicates a doubling time for *E. coli* as 20 minutes. Therefore, after two hours there will be six doubling times. Using the equation 2^n, where n equals the number of generations, and remembering that we started with five *E. coli* cells in the start culture, we rewrite this equation after two hours as 5×2^n, thus, the number of *E. coli* cells in the culture after two hours is $5 \times 2^6 = 320$.

38. The answer is a. (*Levinson, p 44. Ryan, pp 305–306.*) Koch's postulates, formulated by Robert Koch in 1877, were an attempt to determine the cause of infectious disease. Simply stated, they consist of four statements: (1) A specific organism must be isolated from every diseased patient; (2) the organism must be isolated in vitro in pure culture; (3) when inoculated, the pure organism must cause the disease in a healthy, susceptible animal; and (4) the organism must be reisolated from the infected animal.

39. The answer is b. (*Levinson, pp 6–7. Ryan, pp 14–15, 18–21.*) The area indicated by the arrow in the diagram is known as the *periplasmic space,* which is the space between the plasma membrane and the outer membrane. This space contains many hydrolytic enzymes such as alkaline phosphatase, antibiotic-inactivating enzymes such as β-lactamases, and various binding proteins involved in chemotaxis and the active transport of solutes into the cell.

40. The answer is d. (*Levinson, pp 174–175. Ryan, pp 80, 624–628.*) Prions are infectious particles that are composed solely of protein (i.e., they contain no detectable nucleic acid). On the other hand, viruses contain both protein and nucleic acid. Prions give rise to a number of "slow" diseases known as transmissible spongiform encepalopathies such as Creutzfeldt-Jakob disease in humans, bovine spongiform encephalopathy

(BSE) in cows, and scrapie in sheep. Prions are unusually resistant to ultraviolet irradiation, alcohol, formalin, boiling, proteases, and nucleases. They can be inactivated by prolonged exposure to steam autoclaving or IN or 2N NaOH. This has strong implications in the sterilization procedure used for certain medical instruments. The following table is an excellent comparison between conventional viruses and prions.

COMPARISON OF PRIONS AND CONVENTIONAL VIRUSES		
Feature	**Prions**	**Conventional Viruses**
Particle contains nucleic acid	No	Yes
Particle contains protein	Yes, encoded by cellular genes	Yes, encoded by viral genes
Inactivated rapidly by UV light or heat	No	Yes
Appearance in electron microscope	Filamentous rods (amyloid-like)	Icosahedral or helical symmetry
Infection induces antibody	No	Yes
Infection induces inflammation	No	Yes

Reprinted, with permission, from Levinson W, Jawetz E. *Medical Microbiology and Immunology*, 7e. New York: McGraw-Hill, 2002.

41–42. The answers are 41-e, 42-b. (*Levinson, pp 16–17. Ryan, pp 54–57.*) Mutations result from three types of molecular changes, namely, base substitution mutation, frame shift mutation, and transposon or insertion sequences causing mutations. Inversion mutations are caused by insertion sequences (ISs) or IS-like elements. Missense mutation refers to base substitution resulting in a codon that causes a different amino acid to be inserted. Nonsense mutation refers to base substitution generating a termination codon that prematurely stops protein synthesis. Transition mutations are the replacement of a pyrimidine (C, T) by a pyrimidine or a purine (A, G) by a purine. Transversion mutations are the replacement of a purine by a pyrimidine or pyrimidine by a purine.

43–47.   The answers are 43-d, 44-b, 45-c, 46-a, 47-e. *(Levinson, pp 61, 91, 94, 107–108, 140–141. Ryan, pp 198, 220–221, 269–270, 305–307, 484–488.)* The patient in question 43 is infected with *Yersinia pestis* and has bubonic plague. Ceftriaxone or cefotaxime are preferred in the treatment of childhood meningitis because they have the highest activity against the three major causes, namely *Haemophilus influenzae, N. meningitidis,* and *S. pneumoniae.* The patient in question 45 has wool-sorters' disease (inhalation anthrax) from contaminated wool on the farm where he works. Of the third-generation cephalosporins, only ceftazidine is consistently active against *P. aeroginosa.* Finally, the patient in question 47 has acquired a methicillin-resistant *S. aureus* (MRSA) infection, against which vancomycin may be effective. However, *S. aureus* strains are emerging with decreased susceptibility to vancomycin.

48–52.   The answers are 48-e, 49-a, 50-d, 51-b, 52-c. *(Levinson, pp 59–62, 64, 66–70. Ryan, pp 195–198, 201–202, 204, 643–644.)* The antibiotics in these questions have significantly different modes of action. Recent evidence suggests that while penicillin inhibits the final cross-linking of the cell wall, it also binds to penicillin-binding proteins and inhibits certain key enzymes involved in cell-wall synthesis. The mechanism is complex. Amdinocillin, although classified as a penicillin, selectively binds to penicillin-binding protein-2 (PBP-2). Binding to PBP-2 results in aberrant cell-wall elongation and spherical forms, seen when *E. coli,* for example, is exposed to mecillinam.

Because amphotericin binds to sterols (such as ergosterol, a compound of fungal membrane) in the cell membrane, its range of activity is predictable; that is, it is effective against microorganisms that contain sterol in the cell membrane (such as molds, yeasts, and certain amebas). These polyene antibiotics cause reorientation of sterols in the membrane, and membrane structure is altered to the extent that permeability is affected. If sterol synthesis is blocked in fungi, then amphotericin is not effective. This occurs when fungi are exposed to miconazole, another antifungal antibiotic.

Chloramphenicol can be either bacteriocidal or bacteriostatic, depending on the organism. It is bacteriostatic against organisms such as *S. typhi,* but is bacteriocidal against encapsulated organisms that cause meningitis such as *H. influenzae, S. pneumoniae,* and *N. meningitidis.* Bacterial ribosomes are spherical particles. Protein synthesis takes place on the ribosome by a complex process involving various ribosomal subunits, tRNA, and mRNA.

Chloramphenicol, in contrast to the aminoglycosides and tetracycline, attaches to the 50S ribosome subunit. The enzyme peptidyl transferase, found in the 50S subunit, is inhibited. Removal of the inhibition—in this case, chloramphenicol—results in full activity of the enzyme.

Trimethoprim (TMP), a diaminopyrimidine, is a folic acid antagonist. Although TMP is commonly used in combination with sulfa drugs, its mode of action is distinct. TMP is structurally similar to the pteridine portion of dihydrofolate and prevents the conversion of folic acid to tetrahydrofolic acid by inhibition of dihydrofolate reductase. Fortunately, this enzyme in humans is relatively insensitive to TMP.

53–57. The answers are 53-d, 54-c, 55-a, 56-c, 57-b. *(Ryan, pp 251–255.)* The process of PCR is complicated, and its steps are interrelated. A number of steps in the process can markedly affect the results of clinical testing. For example, the detection of amplified products is essential in order to determine whether target nucleic acid was present in the specimen. Product can be detected by staining of the gel that separates the products, Southern blot (a radioactive procedure), or an ELISA-like capture method. A failure of this production step prevents detection of product.

One of the essential parts of the PCR process is the thermal cycling of the reaction. If the reaction is not heated, primer DNA will not hybridize with the target sequences. Nor will the strands reanneal if the mixture is not cooled. Failure of the thermocycler could cause such a problem.

False-positive results are usually due to contamination of the reaction by foreign DNA. In such a case, the foreign DNA sequences are amplified even if the target sequences are not present.

There are a number of reasons why PCR would be falsely negative, but a prime reason is failure to choose the right primer sets. Suboptimum detection of amplified products is another. Ethidium bromide staining of the PCR gel is less sensitive than detection of the products by Southern blot.

58–63. The answers are 58-e, 59-b, 60-b, 61-a, 62-a, 63-d. *(Levinson, pp 6–7, 9, 41–43, 96–97, 100–105, 107, 142. Ryan, pp 19–20, 164, 276, 288–293, 305–307, 329–333, 439–442.)* Bacteria have a variety of components; some are unique to certain genera and species, others are characteristic of all bacteria. All bacteria have peptidoglycan in their cell walls, although the peptidoglycan layer is much thinner in gram-negative than in gram-positive bacteria. In gram-positive bacteria, teichoic acids, polysaccharides, and peptidoglycolipids are covalently attached to the peptidoglycans. While *Mycobacterium* also has peptidoglycan, up to 40% of the cell wall may be a waxy glycolipid that is responsible for the "acid fastness" of *Mycobacterium* and *Nocardia*, an aerobic actinomycete. Bacterial lipopolysaccharide (LPS), also known as *endotoxin*, is found only in gram-negative bacteria. Not only is it a toxic macromolecule, but it also imparts serologic specificity to some gram-negative bacteria such as *Salmonella* and *E. coli*. A core polysaccharide of several sugars is linked to Lipid A by ketodeoxyoctulonate (KDO).

Capsules are found in both gram-positive and gram-negative bacteria. With the exception of those found in *Bacteroides fragilis*, capsules are not in and of themselves toxic but rather are antiphagocytic and are immunologic (or serologic) determinants. Some examples of capsular components are the following:

1. Sialic acid polymers are found in group B *N. meningitidis*. This identical polymer is also found in *E. coli* K1.
2. Group A streptococci in the early stages of growth have hyaluronic acid capsules. The capsule, however, is rapidly destroyed by the organism's own hyaluronidase.
3. *B. anthracis*, the causative agent of anthrax, is the only bacterium to possess a polypeptide capsule that is a polymer of glutamic acid.
4. *S. pneumoniae* type 3 has a repeating polysaccharide capsule of glucose and glucuronic acid.

Virology

Questions

DIRECTIONS: Each question below contains four or more suggested responses. Select the **one best** response to each question.

64. An HIV-positive patient asks you if you can tell him the chances of his progressing to symptomatic AIDS. Which one of the following tests would be most useful?

a. CD4 lymphocyte count
b. HIV antibody test
c. HIV p24 antigen
d. HIV RT PCR
e. Neopterin

65. A 9-year-old male presented with fever and nonspecific symptoms followed by a distinctive rash on the cheeks (slapped cheek). Which of the following viruses may cause this disease and has been associated with transient aplastic crises in persons with sickle cell disease?

a. Herpes simplex
b. Parvovirus
c. Rubella
d. Rubeola
e. Varicella-zoster

66. A 20-year-old female presented to her physician with a low-grade fever, headache, and painful genital lesions. Culture detects herpes simplex virus. Which of the following statements best describes infection with this common human pathogen?

a. Infection with type 1 virus is most common
b. Initial infection usually occurs by intestinal absorption of the virus
c. It can be reactivated by emotional disturbances or prolonged exposure to sunlight
d. It rarely recurs in a host who has a high antibody titer
e. The CNS and visceral organs are usually involved

Questions 67–69

67. The latest and most effective therapy for AIDS patients includes azidothymidine (AZT), dideoxyinosine (DDI), and saquinavir or similar agents. Use of these three drugs would inhibit which of the following viral processes?

a. All membrane synthesis
b. gp120 formation
c. p24 antibody expression
d. Reverse transcriptase, protease
e. RNase, DNase

68. An HIV-positive patient, prior to being treated with AZT, DDI, and saquinavir, has a CD4 lymphocyte count and an HIV RNA viral load test done. Results are as follows:

CD4: 50 CD4 lymphocytes per μL
HIV RNA: 100,000 copies per mL

Which of the following statements best describes this patient?

a. This patient is no longer in danger of opportunistic infection
b. The five-year prognosis is excellent
c. The patient's HIV screening test is most likely negative
d. The patient is not infectious
e. The viral load of 100,000 copies per mL suggests that the patient will respond to triple therapy

69. This HIV-positive patient with a viral load of 100,000 copies of HIV RNA/mL and a total CD4 count of 50 is at an increased risk for a number of infectious diseases. For which of the following diseases is the patient at no more added risk than an immunocompetent host?

a. Herpes simplex virus
b. Kaposi's sarcoma
c. Mycobacterial disease
d. Pneumococcal pneumonia
e. Pneumocystic pneumonia

70. A 19-year-old college student presented at the student health clinic complaining of sore throat, fever, swollen neck lymph nodes, and malaise of several days. Viral capsid antibody (IgM) tested positive, indicating infectious mononucleosis. This potentially debilitating viral disorder is characterized by which of the following statements?

a. Affected persons respond to treatment with the production of heterophil antibodies
b. It is caused by a rhabdovirus
c. It is most prevalent in children less than 14 years old
d. Ribavirin is the treatment of choice
e. The causative pathogen is an Epstein-Barr virus

71. During a medical checkup for a new insurance policy, a 60-year-old grandmother is found to be positive in the ELISA screening test for antibodies against HIV-1. She has no known risk factors for exposure to the virus. Which of the following is the most appropriate next step?

a. Immediately begin therapy with azidothymidine
b. Perform the screening test a second time
c. Request that a blood culture be done by the lab
d. Tell the patient that she is likely to develop AIDS
e. Test the patient for *Pneumocystis carinii* infection

72. Patients in an outbreak of arbovirus disease on a Caribbean island presented with a variety of symptoms, including encephalitis, hemorrhagic fever, or fever with myalgia. Which one of the following is a characteristic of arboviruses?

a. Are closely related to Parvoviruses
b. Are transmitted by insect vectors
c. Are treatable with antiviral chemotherapy
d. Are usually resistant to ether
e. Usually cause symptomatic infection in humans

73. Which one of the following statements best describes interferon's suspected mode of action in producing resistance to influenza virus infection?

a. It stimulates a cell-mediated immunity
b. It stimulates humoral immunity
c. Its direct antiviral action is related to the suppression of messenger RNA formation
d. Its action is related to the synthesis of a protein that inhibits translation or transcription
e. It alters the permeability of the cell membrane so that viruses cannot enter the cell

74. Coronaviruses are recognized by club-shaped surface glycoproteins that are 20 nm long and resemble solar coronas. Which one of the following is a characteristic ability of these viruses?

a. Agglutinate human red blood cells
b. Cause the common cold
c. Grow profusely at 50°C
d. Grow well in the usual cultured cell lines
e. Infect infants more frequently than adults

75. An elderly male patient with known chronic hepatitis B virus (HBV) status suddenly presents with acute hepatitis episodes. Serology confirms HDV co-infection. Which one of the following describes the delta agent?

a. A hepatitis B mutant
b. A defective RNA virus
c. An incomplete hepatitis B virus
d. Hepatitis C
e. Related to hepatitis A virus

76. Which of the following antiviral agents is a purine nucleoside analogue that has shown promise with Lassa fever, influenza A and B, and respiratory syncytial virus (RSV)?

a. Amantadine
b. Acyclovir
c. Ribavirin
d. Rimantadine
e. Vidarabine

77. Echoviruses are cytopathogenic human viruses that mainly infect which of the following?

a. Bladder and urinary tract
b. Blood and lymphatic systems
c. Central nervous system
d. Intestinal tract
e. Respiratory system

78. A newborn infant presented with disseminated vesicular lesions and seemed not to thrive. Herpes simplex virus was suspected, and laboratory confirmation was desired to justify antiviral chemotherapy. The most sensitive test for the diagnosis of herpes simplex (HSV) meningitis in a newborn infant is which of the following?

a. Cerebrospinal fluid (CSF) protein analysis
b. HSV culture
c. HSV IgG antibody
d. HSV polymerase chain reaction
e. Tzanck smear

79. Acute hemorrhagic conjunctivitis (AHC) is a contagious ocular infection characterized by pain, swelling of the eyelids, and subconjunctival hemorrhages. AHC has been reported to be caused by which of the following viruses?

a. Coronavirus
b. Enterovirus
c. Reovirus
d. Respiratory synctial virus
e. Rhinovirus

80. A 10-year-old boy was taken to his pediatrician after experiencing fever, malaise, and anorexia, followed by tender swelling of his parotid glands. Mumps was diagnosed on the clinical presentation. Mumps virus accounts for 10 to 15% of all cases of aseptic meningitis in the United States. Which of the following characterizes infection by this virus?

a. Is apt to recur periodically in many affected persons
b. Is maintained in a large canine reservoir
c. Is preventable by immunization
d. Usually produces severe systemic manifestations
e. Will usually cause mumps orchitis in postpubertal males

81. An otherwise healthy 65-year-old male was in a car accident and broke several ribs on the left side. Approximately 12 days later he developed a painful, well-circumscribed vesicular rash over the left rib cage that persisted for several weeks. The rash is most likely due to which of the following?

a. Primary infection with herpes B virus
b. Primary infection with herpes simplex virus type 1
c. Primary infection with herpes simplex virus type 2
d. Reactivation of latent Epstein-Barr virus
e. Reactivation of latent varicella-zoster virus

82. A 3-year-old child presents at the physician's office with symptoms of coryza, conjunctivitis, low-grade fever, and Koplik's spots. The causative agent of this disease belongs to which one of the following group of viruses?

a. Adenovirus
b. Herpesvirus
c. Paramyxovirus
d. Picornavirus
e. Orthomyxovirus

83. One of the most common sexually transmitted diseases that may lead to cervical carcinoma is caused by which of the following viruses?

a. Adenovirus
b. Cytomegalovirus
c. Epstein-Barr virus
d. Herpes simplex virus
e. Papillomavirus

84. Two siblings, ages 2 and 4, experienced fever, rhinitis, and pharyngitis that resulted in laryngotracheo bronchitis. Both had harsh cough and hoarseness. Which virus is the leading cause of the croup syndrome and, when infecting mammalian cells in culture, will hemabsorb red blood cells?

a. Adenovirus
b. Group B coxsackievirus
c. Parainfluenza virus
d. Rhinovirus
e. Rotavirus

85. Hepatitis E, a recently characterized hepatitis virus, is best described by which of the following statements?

a. It is not a threat to the blood supply
b. It is a major cause of bloodborne hepatitis
c. It is prevalent in North America
d. It is a single-stranded DNA virus
e. The disease resembles hepatitis C

86. Meningitis is characterized by the acute onset of fever and stiff neck. Aseptic meningitis may be caused by a variety of microbial agents. During the initial 24 hours of the course of aseptic meningitis, an affected person's cerebrospinal fluid is characterized by which of the following statements?

a. Decreased protein content
b. Elevated glucose concentration
c. Eosinophilia
d. Lymphocytosis
e. Polymorphonuclear leukocytosis

87. Infection with hepatitis D virus (HDV; delta agent) can occur simultaneously with infection with hepatitis B virus (HBV) or in a carrier of hepatitis B virus, because HDV is a defective virus that requires HBV for its replicative function. What serologic test can be used to determine whether a patient with HDV is an HBV carrier?

a. HBsAg
b. HBc IgM
c. HBeAg
d. HBs IgM
e. HBs IgG

88. A nurse develops clinical symptoms consistent with hepatitis. She recalls sticking herself with a needle approximately four months before, after drawing blood from a patient. Serologic tests for HBsAg, antibodies to HBsAg, and hepatitis A virus (HAV) are all negative; however, she is positive for IgM core antibody. Which of the following characterizes the current health state of the nurse?

a. Does not have hepatitis B
b. Has hepatitis A
c. Has hepatitis C
d. Is in the late stages of hepatitis B infection
e. Is in the "window" (after the disappearance of HBsAg and before the appearance of anti-HBsAg)

89. Eastern equine encephalitis (EEE) virus is associated with a high (50–70%) fatality rate. Control of the disease could be possible by eradication of which one of the following?

a. Birds
b. Fleas
c. Horses
d. Mosquitoes
e. Ticks

90. Rhinovirus is primarily transmitted by which one of the following?

a. Droplet aerosolization
b. Fecal-oral route
c. Fomites
d. Sexual activity
e. Vertical transmission (mother to child)

91. German measles virus (rubella), a common cause of exanthems in children, is best described by which of the following statements?

a. Incubation time is approximately three to four weeks
b. Measles (rubeola) and German measles (rubella) are caused by the same virus
c. Onset is abrupt, with cough, coryza, and fever
d. Specific antibody in the serum does not prevent disease
e. Vesicular rashes are characteristic

92. The presence of Negri inclusion bodies in host cells is characteristic of which of the following?

a. Aseptic meningitis
b. Congenital rubella
c. Infectious mononucleosis
d. Mumps
e. Rabies

93. Kuru is a fatal disease of certain New Guinea natives and is characterized by tremors and ataxia; Creutzfeldt-Jakob disease (CJD) is characterized by both ataxia and dementia. These diseases are thought to be caused by which one of the following?

a. Cell wall–deficient bacteria
b. Environmental toxins
c. Flagellates
d. Prions
e. Slow viruses

94. According to recommendations issued by the U.S. Public Health Service, which of the following statements regarding vaccination against smallpox is true?

a. Children should be vaccinated before they begin school
b. Persons traveling abroad need not be vaccinated
c. Persons who have eczema should be vaccinated soon after diagnosis
d. Persons who have immune deficiencies should be vaccinated every five years
e. Pregnant women should be vaccinated in the first trimester

95. A 35-year-old man developed headache, nausea, vomiting, and sore throat eight weeks after returning from a trip abroad. He eventually refused to drink water and had episodes of profuse salivation, difficulty in breathing, and hallucinations. Two days after the patient died of cardiac arrest, it was learned that he had been bitten by a dog while on his trip. What treatment, if given immediately after the dog bite, could have helped prevent this disease?

a. Bed rest
b. Interleukin 2
c. High-dose acyclovir
d. Broad-spectrum antibiotics
e. Vaccine specific for the etiologic agent

96. A patient who worked in an industrial setting presented to his ophthalmologist with acute conjunctivitis, enlarged and tender preauricular nodes, and early stages of keratitis. The differential diagnosis should include infection with which of the following viruses?

a. Adenovirus
b. Epstein-Barr virus
c. Parvovirus
d. Respiratory syncytial virus
e. Varicella-zoster virus

97. A hospital worker is found to have hepatitis B surface antigen. Subsequent tests reveal the presence of e antigen as well. Which of the following best describes the worker?

a. Is infective and has active hepatitis
b. Is infective but does not have active hepatitis
c. Is not infective
d. Is evincing a biologic false-positive test for hepatitis
e. Has both hepatitis B and hepatitis C

98. Alphavirus causes which one of the following viral diseases?

a. Dengue
b. Marburg virus disease
c. Saint Louis encephalitis
d. Western equine encephalitis
e. Yellow fever

99. Several antiviral compounds have been developed during the last decade. One such compound is ribavirin, a synthetic nucleoside structurally related to guanosine. Ribavirin therapy is FDA-approved for use against which of the following?

a. Group A coxsackievirus
b. Hepatitis B
c. Herpes simplex virus
d. Parvovirus
e. Respiratory syncytial virus

100. An immunocompromised person with a history of seizures had an MRI that revealed a temporal lobe lesion. Brain biopsy results showed multinucleated giant cells with intranuclear inclusions. The most probable cause of the lesion is which of the following?

a. Coxsackievirus
b. Hepatitis C virus
c. Herpes simplex virus
d. *Listeria monocytogenes*
e. Parvovirus

101. A 19-year-old college freshman seeks medical help for symptoms of headache, malaise, fatigue, and sore throat. She admits to attending multiple parties in the dorm. Her physician notes her enlarged lymph nodes and spleen. Which of the following procedures or clinical signs is most specific for the diagnosis of infectious mononucleosis caused by the Epstein-Barr virus?

a. B-cell lymphocyte proliferation
b. Growth in tissue culture cells
c. Heterophile antibodies in serum
d. Laboratory diagnosis based on the presence of "atypical lymphocytes" and EBV-specific antibody
e. Lymphadenopathy and splenomegaly on physical examination

102. A 5-month-old infant, seen in the ER, presents with a fever and persistent cough. Physical examination and a chest x-ray suggest pneumonia. Which of the following is most likely the cause of this infection?

a. Adenovirus
b. Coxsackievirus
c. Respiratory syncytial virus
d. Rhinovirus
e. Rotavirus

103. Which one of the following groups of people may be at increased risk for HIV infection?

a. Factory workers whose coworkers are HIV-positive
b. Foreign service employees who are hospitalized in Zaire for bleeding ulcers
c. Homosexual females
d. Members of a household in which there is a person who is HIV-positive
e. Receptionists at a hospital

104. An obstetrician sees a pregnant patient who was exposed to rubella virus in the eighteenth week of pregnancy. She does not remember getting a rubella vaccination. Which of the following represents the best immediate course of action?

a. Administer rubella immune globulin
b. Administer rubella vaccine
c. Order a rubella antibody titer to determine immune status
d. Reassure the patient because rubella is not a problem until after the thirtieth week
e. Terminate the pregnancy

105. Mad cow disease has been highly publicized in Great Britain. This disease, which is similar to scrapie, is caused by which of the following?

a. A prion
b. A virus
c. A bacterium with a defective cell wall
d. An autoimmune reaction
e. *Rickettsia*

106. A traveler visited a geographic area where hepatitis A was endemic and did not remember to take gamma globulin for passive protection. Four weeks later, he experienced fever, nausea and jaundice, with dark urine. HAV infection was suspected, but all the tests for HAV-IgG and HAV-IgM were nonreactive. Which of the following is a possible cause of this infection?

a. Hepatitis B surface antigen
b. Hepatitis C
c. Hepatitis D
d. Hepatitis E
e. Rotavirus

107. A 70-year-old nursing home patient refused the influenza vaccine and subsequently developed influenza. She died of acute pneumonia one week after contracting the flu. Which of the following is the most common cause of acute postinfluenzal pneumonia?

a. *Escherichia coli*
b. *Klebsiella pneumoniae*
c. *Legionella pneumophilia*
d. *L. monocytogenes*
e. *Staphylococcus aureus*

108. Which of the following viruses is transmitted primarily by the fecal-oral route?

a. Colorado tick fever virus
b. Coxsackievirus
c. Dengue fever virus
d. Saint Louis encephalitis virus
e. Yellow fever virus

109. A husband and wife performed the yearly spring cleaning of their mountain cabin. The wife presented to her physician two weeks later with fever, myalgia, headache, and nausea, followed by progressive pulmonary edema. Which of the following statements best describes the pathogen or disease progression in this patient?

a. Hemolysis is common in infected patients
b. Influenza-like symptoms are followed rapidly by acute respiratory failure
c. It is acquired by inhalation of aerosols of the urine and feces of deer
d. Transmission from human to human is common
e. There is effective antiviral therapy available

110. Which of the following statements best applies to the oncogenes of DNA viruses?

a. They are early viral genes that perform essential viral functions
b. They are cell genes that are expressed during embryonic development
c. They encode a protein that has tyrosine kinase–like activity
d. They are virtually identical to the oncogenes of RNA tumor viruses
e. They are cell genes accidentally incorporated into the viral genome

111. Which one of the following viruses may be a definitive human tumor virus?

a. Epstein-Barr virus (EBV)
b. Herpes simplex virus, type 2 (HSV-2)
c. HIV
d. Papillomavirus
e. Varicella-zoster virus (VZV)

112. Parvovirus infection, the cause of a mild exanthem in children, can also cause which of the following?

a. Acute hemolytic anemia
b. Epidemic acute respiratory disease
c. Gastroenteritis
d. Keratoconjunctivitis
e. Whooping cough–like disease

113. Within the first year of life, an infant exhibited severe hearing loss, ocular abnormalities, and apparent mental retardation. Cytomegalovirus (CMV) infection was detected by viral isolation and PCR. Which one of the following statements best characterizes CMV?

a. It can be transmitted across the placental barrier
b. While a common infection, CMV is almost always symptomatic
c. The CMV can be cultured from red blood cells of infected patients
d. Unlike other viral infections, CMV is not activated by immunosuppressive therapy
e. There is no specific therapy for CMV

114. An outbreak of acute viral gastroenteritis occurred in a child-care center, with several very young children exhibiting nausea, vomiting, and watery, nonbloody diarrhea. Which of the following statements characterizes routine human rotavirus infections?

a. They produce an infection that is seen primarily in adults
b. They produce cytopathic effects in many conventional tissue culture systems
c. They are lipid-containing RNA viruses possessing a double-shelled capsid
d. They can be sensitively and rapidly detected in stools by the enzyme-linked immunosorbent assay (ELISA) technique
e. They have been implicated as a major etiologic agent of infantile respiratory disease

115. Subacute sclerosing panencephalitis (SSPE) is characterized by inflammatory lesions and begins with mild changes in personality, ending with dementia and death. Which of the following statements best describes the disease characteristics?

a. Demyelination is characteristic
b. It is a common event occurring in 1 of 300,000 cases of mumps
c. It is a late CNS manifestation of mumps
d. It is a progressive disease involving both white and gray matter
e. Viral DNA can be demonstrated in brain cells

116. The virus shown in the accompanying electron micrograph contains double-stranded RNA within a double-walled capsid. Which one of the following statements best describes this agent?

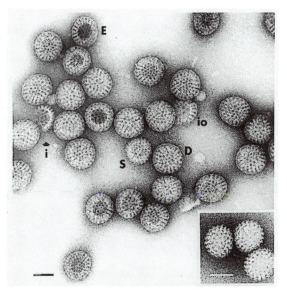

Electron micrograph of a negatively stained preparation of human rotavirus. (D, double-shelled particles; S, single-shelled particles; E, empty capsids; i, fragment of inner shell; io, fragments of a combination of inner and outer shell.) **Inset:** Single-shelled particles obtained by treatment of the viral preparation with sodium dodecyl sulfate. Bars, 50 nm. (*Courtesy of J. Esparza and F. Gil; reproduced, with permission, from Brooks GF, et al. Jawetz's Medical Microbiology, 22e. New York: McGraw-Hill, 2001.*)

a. Early breast-feeding offers no protection to neonates against it
b. It is a major cause of neonatal diarrhea
c. It is readily cultured from the stool of infected persons
d. Maternal antibody does not appear to be protective
e. There are no related animal viruses

117. Helical viruses containing negative sense linear RNA genomes and an outer lipid envelope are most commonly associated with which of the following diseases?

a. Croup
b. Fifth disease
c. Otitis media
d. Rubella
e. Tonsillitis

118. Heat-stable, ether-resistant human viruses containing circular double-stranded DNA genomes are most commonly associated with which of the following?

a. Carcinoma of the lung
b. Condyloma acuminatum
c. Hepatic carcinoma
d. Prostate cancer
e. Rectal polyps

119. Reverse transcriptase is an enzyme found in retroviruses and hepadnaviruses. Which one of the following is a function of the enzyme reverse transcriptase?

a. DNAse activity
b. DNA-dependent RNA polymerase activity
c. RNA-dependent DNA polymerase activity
d. RNA-dependent RNA polymerase activity
e. RNA isomerase activity

120. Several young adults camped in a wilderness area and received multiple mosquito bites. Ten days later, one had a sudden onset of headache, chills, and fever, and became stuporous 48 hours later. He was diagnosed with Saint Louis encephalitis (SLE) and, fortunately, recovered completely. Which of the following best describes SLE?

a. It is transmitted to humans by the bite of an infected tick
b. It is caused by a togavirus
c. It is the major arboviral cause of central nervous system infection in the United States
d. It may present initially with symptoms similar to influenza
e. Laboratory diagnosis is routinely made by cultural methods

121. There is considerable overlap of signs and symptoms seen in congenital and perinatal infections. In a neonate with classic symptoms of congenital CMV infection, which one of the following tests would be most useful in establishing a diagnosis?

a. CMV IgG titer on neonate's serum at birth
b. CMV IgG titer on mother's serum at birth of infant
c. CMV IgM titer on neonate's serum at birth and at one month of age
d. Culture of mother's urine
e. Total IgM on neonate's serum at birth

122. Interferon is produced by cells in tissue culture when the cells are stimulated with which of the following?

a. Botulinum toxin
b. Chlamydiae
c. Gram-positive bacteria
d. Synthetic polypeptides
e. Viruses

123. Viruses have various ways of entering the human body and producing disease. Which of the following descriptions accurately describes the route and mechanism for the virus indicated?

a. Coronaviruses enter the gastrointestinal tract through the mouth and move into the stomach, where they proliferate within mucosal cells to produce peptic ulcers
b. Enteroviruses enter through the mouth, replicate in the pharynx and bowel, and move via the blood to distant target organs (central nervous system)
c. HIV is directly injected into the bloodstream by insects requiring blood for egg development
d. Influenza viruses enter through the respiratory tract, replicate within lymphocytes in the lung, and move via the lymphatic vessels to joints and the CNS to produce muscle aches, stiff joints, and fever
e. Mumps virus enters through abraded skin in the genital area and moves into the testicles of males to produce swelling and sterility

124. A 17-year-old girl presents with cervical lymphadenopathy, fever, and pharyngitis. Infectious mononucleosis is suspected. Which of the following is the most rapid and clinically useful test to make this diagnosis?

a. Antibody to Epstein-Barr nuclear antigen (EBNA)
b. C-reactive protein (CRP)
c. Culture
d. IgG antibody to viral core antigen (VCA)
e. IgM antibody to VCA

125. Which one of the following viruses would be most likely to establish a latent infection?

a. Adenovirus
b. Coxsackievirus group B
c. Influenza virus
d. Measles virus
e. Parvovirus

126. On November 6, a patient had the onset of an illness characterized by fever, chills, headache, cough, and chest pain. The illness lasted one week. On December 5, she had another illness very similar to the first, which lasted six days. She had no flu immunization during this period. Her hemagglutination inhibition (HI) antibody titer to swine flu virus was as follows:

November 6   10
November 30   10
December 20   160
(There was no laboratory error)

Which of the following is the valid conclusion from this data?

a. The patient was ill with swine flu on November 6
b. The patient was ill with swine flu later, and the November 6 illness was due to another pathogen
c. The patient was ill with swine flu on December 20
d. It is impossible to relate either illness with the specific virus

127. Atypical lymphocytosis is most likely to be found in which one of the following diseases?

a. Encephalitis caused by herpes simplex virus (HSV)
b. Chronic hepatitis C
c. Mononucleosis induced by Epstein-Barr virus
d. Parvovirus infection
e. Rotavirus gastroenteritis

128. A tourist who recently returned from a Caribbean cruise suddenly developed arthralgia, a maculopapular rash, and lymphadenopathy with back and bone pain. Which of the following diseases is most likely based on these symptoms?

a. Dengue fever
b. Hepatitis
c. HIV infection
d. Infectious mononucleosis
e. Saint Louis encephalitis

129. A 30-year-old female with a recent history of serious illness requiring surgery developed fever, nausea, and jaundice. Her condition continued as a clinically mild disease, with only minimal elevation of liver enzymes. Hepatitis C (HCV) was diagnosed from laboratory studies. Which one of the following statements best characterizes HCV?

a. Blood products are not tested for antibody to HCV
b. Few cases progress to chronic liver disease
c. HBV but not HCV infections occur in IV drug abusers
d. It is a DNA virus
e. It is the most common cause of posttransfusion hepatitis

Questions 130–133

130. Which of the following markers is usually the first viral marker detected after hepatitis B infection?

a. HBcAg
b. HBeAg
c. HBsAg
d. HBeAb
e. Anti-HBc

131. Which of the following may be the only detectable serological marker during the early convalescent phase of HBV infection (window phase)?

a. HBcAg
b. HBeAg
c. HBsAg
d. HBeAb
e. Anti-HBc

132. Which one of the following markers is closely associated with HBV infectivity and DNA polymerase activity?

a. HBcAg
b. HBeAg
c. HBsAg
d. HBeAb
e. Anti-HBc

133. Which of the following is found within the nuclei of infected hepatocytes and not usually in the peripheral circulation?

a. HBcAg
b. HBeAg
c. HBsAg
d. HBeAb
e. Anti-HBc

Questions 134–138

134. Which one of the following viruses is the leading cause of congenital malformations?

a. Cytomegalovirus
b. Mumps
c. Rabies
d. Respiratory syncytial virus
e. Rhinovirus

135. Orchitis, which may cause sterility, is a possible manifestation of which of the following?

a. Cytomegalovirus
b. Mumps
c. Rabies
d. Respiratory syncytial virus
e. Rhinovirus

136. Which of the following is a leading cause of pneumonia primarily in infants?

a. Cytomegalovirus
b. Mumps
c. Rabies
d. Respiratory syncytial virus
e. Rhinovirus

137. Which of the following causes a fatal encephalitis for which a vaccine is available?

a. Cytomegalovirus
b. Mumps
c. Rabies
d. Respiratory syncytial virus
e. Rhinovirus

138. Traditional vaccination for the common cold is virtually impossible because there are multiple serotypes of which one of the following viruses?

a. Cytomegalovirus
b. Mumps
c. Rabies
d. Respiratory syncytial virus
e. Rhinovirus

Questions 139–143

139. Which of the following is available and effective for hepatitis A?

a. Acyclovir
b. Inactivated virus vaccine
c. Killed virus vaccine
d. Live virus vaccine
e. Recombinant viral vaccine

140. Patients should be vaccinated annually for influenza with which of the following vaccines?

a. Immune serum globulin
b. Inactivated virus vaccine
c. Killed virus vaccine
d. Live virus vaccine
e. Recombinant viral vaccine

141. Which of the following best characterizes the vaccine for measles?

a. Bacterin
b. Inactivated virus vaccine
c. Killed virus vaccine
d. Live virus vaccine
e. Recombinant viral vaccine

142. Which one of the following would be the treatment of choice for HSV infection?

a. Acyclovir
b. Azythromycin
c. Herpes immune globulin
d. Killed virus vaccine
e. Recombinant viral vaccine

143. Which of the following best describes the presently available vaccine for hepatitis B?

a. Inactivated virus vaccine
b. Killed virus vaccine
c. Live virus vaccine
d. Recombinant viral vaccine
e. Synthetic peptide vaccine

Questions 144–148

144. Chickenpox is a common disease of childhood. It is caused by which of the following viruses?

a. Adenovirus
b. Cytomegalovirus
c. Papillomavirus
d. Rotavirus
e. Varicella virus

145. Excluding influenza, which one of the following viruses is a common cause of acute respiratory disease?

a. Adenovirus
b. Cytomegalovirus
c. Papillomavirus
d. Rotavirus
e. Varicella virus

146. Human warts are not only cosmetically unsightly but may lead to cancer of the cervix. They are caused by which one of the following viruses?

a. Adenovirus
b. Cytomegalovirus
c. Papillomavirus
d. Rotavirus
e. Varicella virus

147. A vaccine is available for one of the most common causes of infantile gastroenteritis. However, it has recently been recalled. Which of the following is the virus?

a. Adenovirus
b. Cytomegalovirus
c. Papillomavirus
d. Rotavirus
e. Varicella virus

148. A child has mononucleosis-like symptoms, yet the test for mononucleosis and the EBV titers are negative. Which of the following is one of the causes of heterophile-negative mononucleosis?

a. Adenovirus
b. Coxsackievirus
c. Cytomegalovirus
d. Herpes simplex virus
e. Varicella-zoster virus

Questions 149–153

149. Malaise and fatigue with increased "atypical" lymphocytes and a reactive heterophil antibody test are most commonly caused by which of the following?

a. *Borrelia burgdorferi*
b. Epstein-Barr virus
c. Parvovirus
d. Rubella virus
e. *Toxoplasma*

150. A patient had complement fixation antibody titers against measles virus as follows: acute = 40, convalescent = 80. What conclusion could you make concerning this patient?

a. The patient has a recurrent, acute infection
b. Infection occurred sometime in the past
c. The antibodies could only have been made due to vaccination
d. The patient would be incompletely immune to measles due to lack of CMI immunity
e. An immediate booster shot would be necessary to enhance the patient's protection against measles

151. Burkitt's lymphoma is characterized by elevated "early antigen" tests with a restricted pattern of fluorescence. This disease is caused by which of the following?

a. *B. burgdorferi*
b. Cytomegalovirus
c. Epstein-Barr virus
d. Herpes simplex virus
e. Lymphogranuloma venereum

152. Which of the following viruses may be detected by the polymerase chain reaction (PCR) in a variety of cells of patients with nasopharyngeal carcinoma?

a. Epstein-Barr virus
b. Measles
c. Mumps
d. Parvovirus
e. Rubella

153. This virus causes a mononucleosis-like syndrome caused by a latent herpesvirus; it is often a congenital infection. Large amounts of the virus are excreted in the urine; thus, urine becomes the fluid of choice for diagnosis of this disease. Which of the following is the virus?

a. Cytomegalovirus
b. Epstein-Barr virus
c. HHV-6
d. Norwalk virus
e. Parvovirus

Questions 154–158

Assume you are asked by a resident what the most appropriate specimen is for the detection of a particular virus.

154. Which specimen is best for human papillomavirus?

a. Blood
b. Cervical tissue
c. Skin
d. Synovial fluid

155. Which specimen is best for cytomegalovirus?

a. Blood
b. Cerebrospinal fluid
c. Cervical tissue
d. Skin
e. Synovial fluid

156. Which specimen is best for enterovirus?

a. Blood
b. Cerebrospinal fluid
c. Cervical tissue
d. Skin
e. Synovial fluid

157. Which specimen is best for varicella-zoster virus (VZV)?

a. Blood
b. Cerebrospinal fluid
c. Cervical tissue
d. Skin
e. Synovial fluid

158. Which specimen is best for adenovirus 40/41?

a. Blood
b. Cerebrospinal fluid
c. Cervical tissue
d. Stool
e. Synovial fluid

Questions 159–163

159. Which of the following is transmitted by the fecal-oral route, can be acquired from shellfish, and often causes acute jaundice, diarrhea, and liver function abnormalities?

a. Adenovirus 40/41
b. Astrovirus
c. Hepatitis A virus
d. Norwalk virus
e. Rotavirus

160. Unlike other similar viruses, this virus causes only gastroenteritis. Which of the following is the second most common cause of pediatric gastroenteritis?

a. Adenovirus 40/41
b. Astrovirus
c. Hepatitis A virus
d. Norwalk virus
e. Rotavirus

161. It is difficult to grow in cell culture but can be detected easily by immunologic methods (ELISA). Which of the following is the most common cause of pediatric gastroenteritis?

a. Adenovirus 40/41
b. Astrovirus
c. Hepatitis A virus
d. Norwalk virus
e. Rotavirus

162. It may be detected by ELISA methods or electron microscopy. Which of the following is a common cause of epidemic gastroenteritis, particularly aboard cruise ships and in summer camps?

a. Adenovirus 40/41
b. Astrovirus
c. Hepatitis A virus
d. Norwalk virus
e. Rotavirus

163. It can be transmitted by the fecal-oral route but not by food consumption. Which of the following is a cause of mild gastroenteritis?

a. Adenovirus 40/41
b. Astrovirus
c. Hepatitis A virus
d. Norwalk virus
e. Rotavirus

Questions 164–168

164. IgM antibody to the viral particle is the method of choice for laboratory diagnosis of which one of the following hepatitis viruses?

a. Hepatitis A
b. Hepatitis B
c. Hepatitis C
d. Hepatitis D
e. Hepatitis E

165. This virus belongs to the family of Flaviviruses, and its reservoir is strictly human. Transmission is bloodborne, so the blood supply is routinely screened for which one of the following viruses?

a. Hepatitis A
b. Hepatitis B
c. Hepatitis C
d. Hepatitis D
e. Hepatitis E

166. Vaccination for this hepatic disease is with viral surface antigen and usually provides immunity to which of the following viruses?

a. Hepatitis A
b. Hepatitis B
c. Hepatitis C
d. Hepatitis D
e. Hepatitis E

167. This hepatitis virus is a calicivirus. The reservoir is in pigs, and humans acquire it via the fecal-oral route. Which of the following is the virus?

a. Hepatitis A
b. Hepatitis B
c. Hepatitis C
d. Hepatitis D
e. Hepatitis E

168. This hepatitis virus is a defective virus in that it cannot replicate independently without the presence of hepatitis B virus. Which of the following is the virus?

a. Hepatitis A
b. Hepatitis B
c. Hepatitis C
d. Hepatitis D
e. Hepatitis E

169. Which of the following is the causative agent of a variety of cutaneous warts (plantar, common, and flat) and is associated with cervical neoplasia?

a. Human papillomavirus
b. *Polyomavirus*
c. Subacute sclerosing panencephalitis (SSPE) virus
d. Tick-borne encephalitis virus
e. West Nile virus

170. Recently appearing in the United States, this virus is carried by birds, is transmitted by mosquitoes, and infects humans and horses. Which of the following is the virus?

a. Human papillomavirus
b. *Polyomavirus*
c. Subacute sclerosing panencephalitis (SSPE) virus
d. Tick-borne encephalitis virus
e. West Nile virus

171. Which of the following viruses causes progressive multifocal leukoencephalopathy (PML), a disease causing demyelination in the central nervous system?

a. Human papillomavirus
b. *Polyomavirus*
c. Subacute sclerosing panencephalitis (SSPE) virus
d. Tick-borne encephalitis virus
e. West Nile virus

172. An irritable 18-month-old toddler with fever and blister-like ulcerations on mucous membranes of the oral cavity refuses to eat. The symptoms worsen and then slowly resolve over a period of two weeks. Assuming that the etiological agent was herpes simplex virus type 1, which of the following statements is applicable?

a. Antivirals do not provide any benefit
b. The virus remains latent in the trigeminal ganglia
c. Recurrence is likely to result in a generalized rash
d. Polyclonal B cell activation is a prominent feature
e. The child is at high risk for developing cancer later in life

Questions 173–177

173. This virus is a single-stranded RNA orthomyxovirus. Annual vaccination is necessary because of antigenic drift and shift. Which of the following is the virus?

a. Adenovirus
b. Influenza virus
c. Measles virus
d. Parainfluenza virus
e. Respiratory syncytial virus

174. This virus is a single-stranded RNA paramyxovirus. The rash known as Koplik's spots is pathognomonic Which of the following is the virus?

a. Adenovirus
b. Influenza virus
c. Measles virus
d. Parainfluenza virus
e. Respiratory syncytial virus

175. This virus is the leading cause of bronchiolitis and community-acquired pneumonia in infants. Which of the following is the virus?

a. Adenovirus
b. Influenza virus
c. Measles virus
d. Parainfluenza virus
e. Respiratory syncytial virus

176. This is a paramyxovirus and causes the syndrome known as croup. Which of the following is the virus?

a. Adenovirus
b. Influenza virus
c. Measles virus
d. Parainfluenza virus
e. Respiratory syncytial virus

177. This is a double-stranded DNA virus. It is responsible for 15% of pediatric respiratory infections and 10 to 15% of acute diarrhea in children. Which of the following is the virus?

a. Adenovirus
b. Influenza virus
c. Measles virus
d. Parainfluenza virus
e. Respiratory syncytial virus

Virology

Answers

64. The answer is d. (*Murray—2003, pp 1271–1272. Ryan, pp 614–615.*)
HIV RT PCR, a nucleic acid amplification test for HIV RNA, has recently
been shown to be the most valuable test for (a) monitoring a patient's
progress during triple drug therapy and (b) determining the chances of
progression to AIDS. A viral load of 100,000 to 750,000 copies per mL significantly increases the chance of progression to AIDS within five years.
The other tests listed do not accurately predict progression to AIDS. The
following figure shows the basic structure of HIV, including the enzyme
reverse transcriptase.

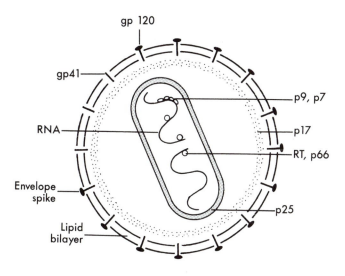

The location of the envelope glycoproteins (gp 120 and gp 124) is shown, as are the
major viral core proteins (p25, p17, p9, and p7). The core protein, p17, is found outside
the viral nucleoid and forms the matrix of the virion. RT indicates reverse transcriptase.

65. The answer is b. *(Murray—2002, pp 506–508. Ryan, pp 522–523.)* Parvovirus B19 is the causative agent of erythema infectiosum (fifth disease). It is associated with transient aplastic crisis in persons with hereditary hemolytic anemia. In adults, it is also associated with polyarthralgia (and fetal loss in pregnant women). Serology detects specific IgM antibody to Parvovirus.

66. The answer is c. *(Gilligan, pp 47–50. Murray—2002, pp 480–482. Ryan, p 558.)* The initial infection by herpes simplex virus is often inapparent and occurs through a break in the skin or mucous membranes, such as in the eye, throat, or genitals. Latent infection often persists at the initial site despite high antibody titers. Recurrent disease can be triggered by temperature change, emotional distress, and hormonal factors. Type 1 herpes simplex virus is usually, but not exclusively, associated with ocular and oral lesions; type 2 is usually, but not exclusively, associated with genital and anal lesions. Type 2 infection is more common. In addition to mucocutaneous infections, the CNS and occasionally visceral organs can be involved.

67–69. The answers are 67-d, 68-e, 69-d. *(Levinson, pp 291–293. Murray—2002, pp 586–587. Ryan, pp 615–616.)* The advent of triple therapy, or a therapeutic "cocktail," has had a marked effect on AIDS patients. The combination of drugs works together as reverse transcriptive inhibitors and a protease inhibitor. Patients improve rapidly, their CD4 lymphocyte counts increase, and their HIV viral loads are drastically reduced, often to less than 50 copies per mL. On the other hand, an untreated HIV-positive patient with a low CD4 and a high viral load (a) is at increased risk of opportunistic infection and (b) has a much greater chance of developing AIDS than if the viral load was less than 10,000. The patient is infectious and his HIV antibody screening test will be positive. The high viral load, however, is not a predictor of response to therapy. Many patients with high viral loads do very well on triple therapy, although resistance to one or more of the agents may subsequently occur. A low CD4 count does not predict progression to AIDS but does indicate increased chance of opportunistic infection such as those listed. Kaposi's sarcoma, which has been linked to herpesvirus type 8, pneumocystis, and mycobacterial disease are three of the most prevalent opportunistic infections. While HIV-positive patients contract pneumococcal pneumonia, they are probably at no more risk than the general population, as protection against pneumococcal disease is linked to the presence of anticapsular antibody.

70. The answer is e. *(Murray—2002, pp 487–491. Ryan, pp 571–573.)* All of Koch's postulates have been verified for the relationship between infectious mononucleosis and Epstein-Barr virus, a herpesvirus. However, the relationship between this virus and Burkitt's lymphoma, sarcoid, and systemic lupus erythematosus (SLE) is less clear. Infectious mononucleosis is most common in young adults (14 to 18 years of age) and is very rare in young children. There is no specific treatment. Heterophil antibody titer is helpful in diagnosis, but is not expressed as a function of clinical recovery.

71. The answer is b. *(Brooks, pp 525–526. Levinson, pp 292–293. Murray—2002, pp 585–586. Ryan, pp 614–615.)* The standard screening test for HIV antibody detection is the enzyme-linked immunosorbant test (ELISA). It is well standardized and available in kit format for relative ease of use in laboratories. As a screening test, however, some false-positive and false-negative results may occasionally be obtained. The standard practice, therefore, is to always perform a second ELISA test before reporting any test result. In fact, before any final report in HIV diagnosis is sent out, a confirming test (western blot test, in most cases) will need to be performed. HIV culture is not routinely done. No evidence of *P. carinii* was noted in the history. Until confirmed, no AZT use is justified and, certainly, no suggestion of AIDS development would be made on the basis of screening test results.

72. The answer is b. *(Murray—2002, pp 557–564. Ryan, pp 587–593.)* Arboviruses (arthropod-borne viruses) may or may not be surrounded by a lipid envelope, although most are inactivated by lipid solvents such as ether and may contain either double-stranded or single-stranded RNA. Physicochemical studies have demonstrated a great heterogeneity among these viruses. Arboviruses cause disease in vertebrates; in humans, encephalitis is a frequent arbovirus illness. Most human infections with arbovirus, however, are asymptomatic.

73. The answer is d. *(Levinson, pp 201–202. Murray—2002, pp 446–447. Ryan, p 104.)* Interferon is a protein produced by cells in response to a viral infection or certain other agents. Entering uninfected cells, interferon causes production of a second protein that alters protein synthesis. As a result of inhibition of either translation or transcription, new viruses are not assembled following infection of interferon-protected cells.

74. The answer is b. *(Brooks, pp 488–491. Murray—2002, pp 611–612. Ryan, p 511.)* Coronaviruses, discovered in 1965, are thought to be a major agent of the common cold, especially in older children and adults. The virion is known to contain RNA, but other elements of its structure are unclear. At 34°C, viral multiplication is profuse; however, infectivity is greatly reduced at higher temperatures or following extended incubation. Rhinoviruses (picornaviruses) are the other major cause of the common cold.

75. The answer is b. *(Levinson, pp 264–265. Murray—2002, pp 591–592. Ryan, pp 550–551.)* The delta agent was first described in 1977 and has recently been shown to be a defective RNA virus that requires HBsAg for replication. It is found most often in persons who have multiple parenteral exposures—for example, intravenous (IV) drug abusers, hemophiliacs, and multiply transfused patients.

76. The answer is c. *(Brooks, p 348. Murray—2002, pp 446–447. Ryan, pp 209–210.)* As an IV agent, ribavirin is effective against Lassa fever in the first week of onset of the disease. It may also be administered as an aerosol that is quite useful in infants with RSV. Unlike amantadine, which is efficacious only with influenza A, ribavirin has activity against both influenza A and influenza B if administered by aerosol in the first 24 hours of onset.

77. The answer is d. *(Brooks, pp 428–429. Murray—2002, pp 517–518. Ryan, pp 537–539.)* Echoviruses were discovered accidentally during studies on poliomyelitis. They were named *enteric cytopathogenic human orphan* (ECHO) viruses because, at the time, they had not been linked to human disease and thus were considered "orphans." Echoviruses now are known to infect the intestinal tract of humans; they also can cause aseptic meningitis, febrile illnesses, and the common cold. Echoviruses range in size from 24 to 30 nm in diameter and contain a core of RNA.

78. The answer is d. *(Ryan, pp 561–562. Brooks, pp 376–377. Murray— 2002, pp 482–483.)* HSV meningitis or encephalitis is difficult to diagnose by laboratory tests, as there is a low titer of virus present in the cerebrospinal fluid. Neonatal HSV infects the child during the birth process. While culture, Tzanck smear, and even antibody tests may be useful in adults, particularly those with HSV-rich lesions, they are not useful for CSF testing. Only PCR is sensitive enough to detect HSV DNA in the CSF. Once diagnosed rapidly, HSV encephalitis or meningitis can be treated with acyclovir.

79. The answer is b. *(Brooks, p 429. Levinson, p 254. Murray—2002, p 518.)* Enterovirus and coxsackievirus A can be recovered from conjunctival scrapings of patients with acute hemorrhagic conjunctivitis (AHC) during the first three days of illness. Isolation rates are somewhat higher for enterovirus than for coxsackievirus. Less than 5% of throat swab or fecal specimens have been positive for either virus. Echovirus 70 is the chief cause of this disease.

80. The answer is c. *(Brooks, pp 480–481. Levinson, pp 241–242. Murray—2002, pp 530–532. Ryan, pp 514–515.)* Much of the public's understanding of mumps is based on suppositions that are without any scientific basis. For example, natural mumps infection confers immunity after a single infection, even if the infection was a unilateral, not a bilateral, parotitis. Also, sterility from mumps orchitis is not ensured; only 20% of males older than 13 years of age develop orchitis. The majority of patients with mumps do not develop systemic manifestations. In fact, some do not develop parotitis. Last, the virus is maintained exclusively in human populations; canine reservoirs are not known. The mumps vaccine is a live attenuated virus vaccine derived from chick-embryo tissue culture.

81. The answer is e. *(Brooks, pp 378–379. Levinson, pp 225–226. Murray—2002, pp 484–486. Ryan, pp 563–565.)* This is a classic description for a reactivation of varicella-zoster viral latent infection. Many initial infections with VZV are subclinical and result in latent infections in sensory ganglion nerve tissue. Varicella (chickenpox) is mild and highly contagious in children. Zoster (shingles) is a sporadic, incapacitating illness seen in adults. Treatment may include acyclovir or famciclovir. Herpes B virus infections occur primarily in monkeys. HSV primary infections are most often subclinical and occur primarily in children. Epstein-Barr virus (infectious mononucleosis) persists in latent infections in B lymphocytes.

82. The answer is c. *(Brooks, pp 476–477. Levinson, pp 240–241. Murray—2002, pp 527–528. Ryan, pp 517–518.)* Koplik's spots are pathognomonic for measles. The measles virus is a paramyxovirus. In industrialized countries, vaccination has reduced the importance of this childhood infection (although U.S. incidence increased in 1989 and 1990). In developing countries, however, measles is a major killer of young children. In America, most states now require proof of immunity before school enrollment, and this has reduced the incidence of disease.

83. The answer is e. *(Brooks, pp 511–513. Levinson, pp 232–233. Murray—2002, pp 460–462. Ryan, p 619.)* Human papillomavirus (HPV) is the cause of genital warts. It is one of the most pervasive of all the sexually transmitted diseases. There is no specific cure or vaccine. There are multiple serotypes of papillomavirus, and some serotypes are linked to cervical cancer. New techniques for molecular diagnosis of HPV show promise for rapid and sensitive detection and perhaps more aggressive treatment. Herpes simplex virus type II (HSV-II) was originally thought to be etiologically involved, but is now not considered so. HSV-II evidence came primarily from serological data.

84. The answer is c. *(Brooks, pp 476–478. Levinson, pp 243–244. Murray—2002, pp 529–530. Ryan, pp 506–507.)* Parainfluenza viruses are important causes of respiratory diseases in infants and young children. The spectrum of disease caused by these viruses ranges from a mild febrile cold to croup, bronchiolitis, and pneumonia. Parainfluenza viruses contain RNA in a nucleocapsid encased within an envelope derived from the host cell membrane. Infected mammalian cell culture will hemabsorb red blood cells owing to viral hemagglutinin on the surface of the cell.

85. The answer is a. *(Brooks, p 408. Levinson, p 265. Murray—2002, p 593.)* Hepatitis E is a newly recognized single-stranded RNA virus in the calicivirus family. Epidemics have been observed in Asia, Africa, India, and Mexico. Like

HAV, it is enterically transmitted, but there is no vaccine available nor is there a routine detection test. Chronic liver disease does not occur, and because it is not bloodborne, it is of no threat to the blood supply.

86. The answer is e. *(Brooks, p 625.)* Aseptic meningitis is characterized by a pleocytosis of mononuclear cells in the cerebrospinal fluid; polymorphonuclear cells predominate during the first 24 hours, but a shift to lymphocytes occurs thereafter. The cerebrospinal fluid of affected persons is free of culturable bacteria and contains normal glucose and slightly elevated protein levels. Peripheral white blood cell counts usually are normal. Although viruses are the most common cause of aseptic meningitis, spirochetes, chlamydiae, and other microorganisms also can produce the disease.

CSF findings	Bacterial: pressure ↑, polys ↑, proteins ↑, glucose ↓.
	Viral: pressure normal / ↑, lymphs ↑, proteins normal, glucose normal.
	TB/fungal: pressure ↑, lymphs ↑, proteins ↑, glucose ↓.

87. The answer is c. *(Brooks, pp 412–413.)* In a chronic HBV carrier, there would be no HB core IgM antibody, whereas it would be present in a new HBV infection. The HBe antigen could be present in either an HBV carrier or in acute infection. HBsAg would be present in either a new infection or in the carrier state, while HBsAb would not be present in either case.

88. The answer is e. *(Brooks, p 412. Levinson, pp 261–262. Murray—2002, pp 600–601. Ryan, p 549.)* In a small number of patients with acute hepatitis B infection, HBsAg can never be detected. In others, HBsAg becomes negative before the onset of the disease or before the end of the clinical illness. In such patients with acute hepatitis, hepatitis B virus infection may be established only by the presence of anti–hepatitis B core IgM (anti–HBc IgM), a rising titer of anti-HBc, or the subsequent appearance of anti-HBsAg.

INTERPRETATION OF HBV SEROLOGIC MARKERS IN PATIENTS WITH HEPATITIS*			
Assay Results			
HBsAg	Anti-HBs	Anti-HBc	Interpretation
Positive	Negative	Negative	Early acute HBV infection. Confirmation is required to exclude nonspecific reactivity.
Positive	(±)	Positive	HBV infection, either acute or chronic. Differentiate with IgM anti-HBc. Determine level of replicative activity (infectivity) with HBeAg or HBV DNA.
Negative	Positive	Positive	Indicates previous HBV infection and immunity to hepatitis B.
Negative	Negative	Positive	Possibilities include: HBV infection in remote past; "low-level" HBV carrier; "window" between disappearance of HBsAg and appearance of anti-HBs; or false-positive or nonspecific reaction. Investigate with IgM anti-HBc, challenge with HBsAg vaccine, or both. When present, anti-HBe helps validate the anti-HBc reactivity.
Negative	Negative	Negative	Another infectious agent, toxic injury to liver, disorder of immunity, hereditary disease of the liver, or disease of the biliary tract.
Negative	Positive	Negative	Vaccine-type response.

*Modified and reproduced, with permission, from Hollinger FB. Hepatitis B virus. In: Fields BN et al (ed). Fields Virology, 3e. Lippincott-Raven, 1996.

89. The answer is d. (*Brooks, p 445. Levinson, pp 268–269.*) Eastern equine encephalitis (EEE) is a severe disease usually seen in the summer months when *Aedes* mosquitoes are prevalent. In 1996 and 1997, there were several outbreaks in the northeastern United States. Control of EEE is a function of mosquito eradication. Horses and humans are accidental hosts. If the patient survives, the CNS sequelae are usually severe. While draining of swamps helps, other measures to eliminate mosquitoes, such as spraying, are the most effective.

90. The answer is c. *(Brooks, pp 430–431. Levinson, pp 254–255. Murray—2002, p 520.)* Rhinovirus is a major cause of the common cold. The primary mode of transmission is the contact of contaminated hands, fingers, or fomites with the conjunctiva or nasal epithelium. While several studies have shown no evidence of aerosol transmission, a study by Dick and associates in 1986 did show aerosol transmission can occur. This is not, however, the main mode of transmission.

91. The answer is c. *(Brooks, pp 484–486. Levinson, pp 244–245. Murray—2002, pp 565–567. Ryan, pp 519–520.)* Measles (rubeola) is an acute, highly infectious disease characterized by a maculopapular rash. German measles (rubella) is an acute, febrile illness characterized by a rash as well as suboccipital lymphadenopathy. Incubation time is nine full days after exposure. Onset is abrupt and symptoms mostly catarrhal. Koplik's spots, pale, bluish-white spots in red areolas, can frequently be observed on the mucous membranes of the mouth and are pathognomonic for measles.

92. The answer is e. *(Brooks, p 495. Levinson, pp 245–246. Murray—2002, pp 449–450. Ryan, p 599.)* The definitive diagnosis of rabies in humans is based on the finding of Negri bodies, which are cytoplasmic inclusions in the nerve cells of the spinal cord and brain, especially in the hippocampus. Negri bodies are eosinophilic and generally spherical in shape; several may appear in a given cell. Negri bodies, although pathognomonic for rabies, are not found in all cases of the disease.

93. The answer is d. *(Brooks, pp 499–500. Levinson, pp 283–285. Murray—2002, pp 607–610. Ryan, pp 625–627.)* Kuru and CJD are similar but not identical diseases with very different epidemiology. Kuru is prevalent among certain tribes in New Guinea who practiced ritual cannibalism by eating the brains of the departed. CJD is found worldwide and has been transmitted by corneal transplants and in pituitary hormone preparations. There is some association between CJD and mad cow disease in England. Prions are unconventional self-replicating proteins, sometimes called *amyloid*. It is now thought that CJD, kuru, and animal diseases such as scrapie, visna, and bovine spongiform encephalopathy (mad cow disease) are caused by prions.

94. The answer is b. (*Brooks, p 398. Levinson, pp 229–230.*) Routine vaccination of infants and children for smallpox has been discontinued in the United States, both because the risk of contracting the disease is so low and because the complications of smallpox vaccination, including generalized vaccinia eruption, postvaccinal encephalitis, and fetal vaccinia, are significant. Owing to the extremely effective eradication of smallpox worldwide by the World Health Organization, U.S. citizens traveling abroad no longer require vaccination. Pregnancy, immune deficiencies, and eczema and other chronic dermatitides are contraindications to smallpox vaccination.

95. The answer is e. (*Brooks, pp 495–497. Levinson, pp 245–247. Murray— 2002, pp 552–554. Ryan pp 597–600.*) Rabies is caused by a rhabdovirus (contains negative sense RNA, helical structure). The virus has a wide host of warm-blooded animals, including humans. The virus is widely distributed in the infected animals, with high levels in saliva. Street viruses (freshly isolated strains) have long incubation periods, leading to eventual viral infection of the CNS. Essentially, all organs are infected, giving rise to the described symptoms. Fixed (mutant) virus strains do not grow in neural tissue. Because of the long incubation period (weeks), active treatment (inactivated vaccine) and passive treatment (human or horse immune globulin) are used to prevent disease. If symptoms appear, essentially 100% fatality results. All other answer options are ineffective against rabies disease.

96. The answer is a. (*Brooks, p 367. Levinson, pp 231–232. Murray—2002, p 472.*) Adenovirus type 8 is associated with epidemic keratoconjunctivitis, while adenovirus types 3 and 4 are often associated with "swimming pool conjunctivitis." There are also reports of nosocomial conjunctivitis with adenovirus. Herpes simplex virus can infect the conjunctiva and is among the most common causes of blindness in North America and Europe.

97. The answer is a. (*Brooks, p 404. Levinson, pp 261–262. Murray—2002, pp 600–601. Ryan, pp 547–549.*) The e antigen is related to the hepatitis B virus and is associated with viral replication (Dane particle). Possession of the e antigen suggests active disease and, thus, an increased risk of transmission of hepatitis to others. HBsAg and e antigen are components of hepatitis B only and are not shared by other hepatitis viruses.

98. The answer is d. (*Brooks, p 442. Levinson, p 268. Murray—2002, p 558. Ryan, p 586.*) Saint Louis encephalitis, yellow fever, and dengue are caused by Flaviviruses. Western equine encephalitis is caused by an alphavirus. Laboratory diagnosis is usually made by demonstration of a fourfold rise in specific antibody titer in paired sera, although viruses may be isolated in specialist laboratories.

99. The answer is e. *(Brooks, pp 348–349. Levinson, p 211. Murray—2002, pp 446–447. Ryan, pp 209–210.)* Ribavirin is effective to varying degrees against several RNA- and DNA-containing viruses in vitro. It has been approved for aerosol treatment of respiratory syncytial virus infections in infants. Intravenous administration has proved effective in treating Lassa fever.

100. The answer is c. *(Brooks, p 376. Murray—2002, pp 478–482. Ryan, pp 559–560.)* Herpes simplex virus causes primary and recurrent disease. The typical skin lesion is a vesicle that contains virus particles in serous fluid. Giant multinucleated cells are typically found at the base of the herpesvirus lesion. Encephalitis, which usually involves the temporal lobe, has a high mortality rate. Severe neurologic sequelae are seen in surviving patients. PCR amplification of viral DNA from CSF has replaced viral isolation.

101. The answer is d. *(Brooks, pp 387–388. Levinson, p 228. Murray—2002, pp 491–492. Ryan, pp 571–572.)* Contact with infected secretions such as saliva can result in infection with EBV, thus the term *kissing disease*. Laboratory diagnosis of EBV-induced infectious mononucleosis is usually determined by presence of atypical lymphocytes, heterophile antibodies, or specific antiviral antibodies such as VCA (viral capsid antibody).

102. The answer is c. *(Brooks, pp 478–479. Levinson, pp 242–243. Murray—2002, pp 532–533. Ryan, pp 504–506.)* Respiratory syncytial virus (RSV) is the most important cause of pneumonia and bronchiolitis in infants. The infection is localized to the respiratory tract. The virus can be detected rapidly by immunofluorescence on smears of respiratory epithelium. In older children, the infection resembles the common cold. Aerosolized ribavirin is recommended for severely ill hospitalized infants.

103. The answer is b. *(Brooks, pp 526–528. Levinson, pp 289–294. Murray—2002, pp 585–587. Ryan, pp 609–610.)* Many believe that casual contact with patients who are HIV-positive increases the risk of acquiring the disease. This is not the case. It is also clear that homosexual females have a low rate of HIV acquisition. Because a substantial portion of the blood supply in Central African countries is HIV-infected, hospitalization is risky, particularly if transfusion is necessary.

104. The answer is c. *(Brooks, p 485. Levinson, p 245. Murray—2002, p 567. Ryan, pp 519–520.)* The highest risk of fetal infection with rubella occurs during the first trimester. In seronegative patients, the risk of infection exceeds 90%. However, before other measures (such as termination of pregnancy) are considered, a rubella immune status must be performed. A rubella titer of 1:10 is protective.

105. The answer is a. *(Brooks, p 500. Levinson, p 285. Murray—2002, p 608. Ryan, pp 627–628.)* Mad cow disease is related to both scrapie in sheep and bovine spongiform encephalopathy virus. The fear in Great Britain is the potential for acquiring Creutzfeldt-Jakob disease, which is a slowly progressive neurodegenerative disease. Theoretically, such acquisition could be through ingestion of beef from infected cows. A prion consists of protein material without nucleic acid. While related to a virus, a prion is a proteinaceous infectious particle that replicates within cells.

106. The answer is d. *(Brooks, p 408. Levinson, p 265. Murray—2002, p 604. Ryan, pp 552–553.)* Hepatitis E virus (HEV) is a single-stranded RNA virus. It is transmitted enterically, and the disease is often referred to as *enteric hepatitis C.* There is no test for HEV routinely available. Diagnosis is clinical and is also one of exclusion. Rotavirus primarily affects children and not adults.

107. The answer is e. *(Brooks, p 465. Murray—2002, p 541. Ryan, p 501.)* S. aureus is the most common cause of postinfluenzal secondary bacterial pneumonia. It most often affects the elderly, although patients of any age may be afflicted. The pneumococcus as well as group A streptococci and *Haemophilus influenzae* may also cause pneumonia.

108. The answer is b. *(Brooks, p 422. Levinson, p 250. Murray—2002, p 511. Ryan, p 531.)* Saint Louis encephalitis virus is spread by mosquitoes and causes a severe encephalitis with a near 10% fatality rate. Colorado tick fever, spread by the wood tick, causes fever, headache, retroorbital pain, and severe myalgia. Fever and jaundice characterize yellow fever, a life-threatening disease spread by mosquitoes. Following fever, headache, myalgias, and photophobia, the symptoms progress to the liver, kidney, and heart. Mortality rate is high. Dengue fever shares the same mosquito vector as yellow fever. Classic dengue fever (breakbone fever) includes flulike symptoms. Severe muscle and joint (breakbone) pain occurs. Coxsackievirus (as well as poliovirus and echoviruses) is spread by the fecal-oral route.

109. The answer is b. (*Levinson, p 197.*) In 1993, an outbreak of a fatal respiratory disease occurred in the southwestern United States. This disease is caused by a hantavirus endemic in deer mice. The mortality rate is 60%. Ribavirin has been used but is not effective. A vaccine is not available. Person-to-person transmission has been reported in South American outbreaks but is uncommon.

110. The answer is a. (*Brooks, et al., pp 501–503. Levinson, pp 274–275. Murray—2002, pp 574–575. Ryan, pp 110–112.*) DNA tumor viruses encode viral oncoproteins that are important to viral replication but also affect cellular growth control pathways. Most RNA tumor viruses belong to the retrovirus family, carrying a reverse transcriptase enzyme (RNA-dependent DNA polymerase) that is responsible for contructing a DNA copy of the viral RNA genome. Direct-transforming RNA oncoviruses carry an oncogene of cellular origin, whereas weakly oncogenic RNA viruses have no oncogene and produce leukemias after long incubation periods by indirect mechanisms.

ASSOCIATION OF VIRUSES WITH HUMAN CANCERS.*		
Virus Family	**Virus**	**Human Cancer**
Papovaviridae	Human papillo-maviruses	Genital tumors Squamous cell carcinoma Oropharyngeal carcinoma
Herpesviridae	EB virus	Nasopharyngeal carcinoma African Burkitt's lymphoma B-cell lymphoma
Hepadnaviridae	Hepatitis B virus	Hepatocellular carcinoma
Retroviridae	HTL virus	Adult T cell leukemia
Flaviviridae	Hepatitis C virus	Hepatocellular carcinoma

*Candidate human tumor viruses include human herpesvirus 8, additional types of papillomaviruses, and human and simian polyomaviruses.

Reprinted, with permission, from Brooks GF et al. Jawetz's Medical Microbiology, 22e. New York: McGraw-Hill, 2001.

111. The answer is d. (*Brooks, pp 512–513. Levinson, pp 232–233. Murray—2002, pp 460–462.*) Only two human viruses have been confirmed as human tumor viruses. They include human T cell lymphotrophic/leukemia virus (HTLV) and papillomavirus. Others, such as EBV, HSV, and hepatitis B and C, have been implicated as tumor viruses. The virus that causes chickenpox and shingles (VZV) is not know to be oncogenic.

112. The answer is a. (*Brooks, pp 358–359. Levinson, pp 233–234. Murray—2002, pp 507–508. Ryan, pp 522–523.*) Adenoviruses are widespread and cause a variety of respiratory and gastrointestinal clinical problems. Many of the "viral sore throats" among young people living in close quarters are due to adenovirus. Parvovirus B19, not adenovirus, causes acute hemolytic anemia.

113. The answer is a. (*Brooks, pp 384–385. Levinson, pp 226–227. Murray—2002, pp 493–494. Ryan, pp 567–568.*) Although infection with cytomegalovirus (CMV) is common, it only rarely causes clinically apparent disease. Lesions characteristic of infection with CMV are found in up to 10% of stillborn babies; however, CMV, which can be transmitted transplacentally, usually is not the cause of death. Children and adults with immunosuppressive problems are susceptible to active disease. In severely immunodeficient patients such as those with AIDS, CMV ocular disease may occur. The patient suffers blurring of vision or vision loss, and ophthalmic examination reveals large yellowish-white areas with flame-shaped hemorrhages. Ganciclovir is now licensed for treatment of CMV retinitis in AIDS patients.

114. The answer is d. (*Brooks, pp 435–437. Levinson, pp 255–256. Murray—2002, pp 547–548. Ryan, pp 578–580.*) Rotaviruses were initially identified by direct electron microscopy (EM) of duodenal mucosa of infants with gastroenteritis. Subsequent studies in several countries have shown them to be the cause of 30 to 40% of cases of acute diarrhea in infants. They are non-lipid-containing RNA viruses with a double-shelled capsid. Although the virus has been serially propagated in human fetal intestinal organ cultures, cytopathic changes are minimal or absent; multiplication is detected by immunofluorescence. Numerous methods for rotavirus antigen detection, including radioimmunoassay, counterimmunoelectrophoresis, and enzyme-linked immunosorbent assay, have been developed and found to be about as effective as EM.

115. The answer is d. *(Brooks, p 483. Levinson, p 283. Murray—2002, p 528. Ryan, pp 517–518.)* SSPE is a late and rare manifestation of measles. It is a progressive encephalitis involving both white and gray matter. Demyelination is seen only at an advanced stage of the disease in a few cases. In 1985, viral RNA was demonstrated in brain cells from a patient with SSPE by the use of in situ hybridization.

116. The answer is b. *(Brooks, pp 435–437. Levinson, pp 255–256. Murray—2002, pp 547–548. Ryan, pp 578–580.)* Rotavirus is a viral entity that is similar to Nebraska calf diarrhea virus and is thought to be a major cause of acute diarrhea in newborn infants. Three-quarters of all adults have antibodies against rotavirus; passive transfer of these antibodies to the baby, especially through the colostrum, seems to be protective. Although vaccination would be expected to be of little use to the neonate, it might effectively immunize pregnant mothers.

117. The answer is a. *(Brooks, pp 476–478. Levinson, pp 243–244. Murray—2002, pp 529–530. Ryan, pp 506–507.)* Both mumps and measles are well-recognized paramyxovirus infections. This group also includes parainfluenza virus, which causes laryngotracheobronchitis (croup) in children, and respiratory syncytial virus, which can cause bronchiolitis in infants. Paramyxoviruses have glycoprotein spikes that extend their lipid membrane and are responsible for hemagglutination activities.

118. The answer is b. *(Brooks, pp 318, 513. Levinson, pp 232–233. Murray—2002, p 461. Ryan, p 902.)* Papillomavirus infects the skin or mucosa and causes benign tumors. The lesion is termed *condyloma acuminatum.* These tumors may undergo malignant conversion and become squamous cell carcinomas. Classification of the human papillomavirus is done by DNA hybridization, and, to date, 46 types have been recognized. Some types, such as 16 and 18, are more frequently associated with carcinoma, while others, such as 6 and 11, are associated with benign tumors or warts.

119. The answer is c. *(Brooks, p 408. Levinson, p 260. Murray—2002, p 596. Ryan, p 545.)* The replication of a retroviral genome is dependent on the reverse transcriptase enzyme, which performs a variety of functions. It builds a complementary strand of DNA for the viral RNA template; it builds a second DNA strand complementary to the previous DNA; it degrades the original RNA, leaving a DNA-DNA duplex; and, finally, it is responsible for integrating the new viral DNA hybrid into the host genome.

120. The answer is c. (*Brooks, pp 445–447. Levinson, pp 268–269. Murray—2002, pp 562–563. Ryan, p 591.*) Saint Louis encephalitis virus has structural and biologic characteristics in common with other Flaviviruses. It is the most important arboviral disease in North America. Saint Louis encephalitis virus was first isolated from mosquitoes in California. Patients who contract the disease usually present with one of three clinical manifestations: febrile headache, aseptic meningitis, or clinical encephalitis.

121. The answer is c. (*Brooks, p 383. Levinson, pp 226–227. Murray—2002, p 496. Ryan, p 568.*) (See figure below.) Presently, cytomegalovirus (CMV) is the most common cause of congenital and perinatal viral infections. Culture of the virus is a sensitive diagnostic technique; in the case of a neonate with classic symptoms, serum samples from the mother and neonate are obtained at birth. The IgM antibody titer in the infant's serum should be higher than the mother's titer, but they may be similar. For this reason, another sample from the infant at one month of age is tested simultaneously with the initial sample. The results should indicate a rise in IgM titer. Measurement of total IgM in the infant's sera at birth is nonspecific and may show false-negative and false-positive reactions.

Cytomegalovirus-infected human embryonic fibroblasts stained with fluorescein-labeled monoclonal antibody to early nuclear antigen (×1000).

122. The answer is e. *(Brooks, pp 350–351. Levinson, pp 201–202. Murray—2002, pp 131–133. Ryan, pp 104, 212.)* Interferon is a protein that alters cell metabolism to inhibit viral replication. It induces the formation of a second protein that interferes with the translation of viral messenger RNA. Production of interferon has been demonstrated when cells in tissue culture are challenged with viruses, rickettsiae, endotoxin, or synthetic double-stranded polynucleotides. Interferon confers species-specific, not virus-specific, protection for cells.

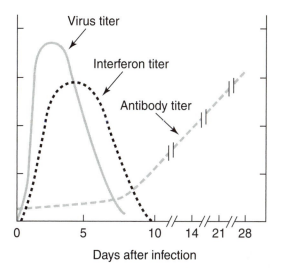

Illustration of kinetics of interferon and antibody synthesis after respiratory viral infection. The temporal relationships suggest that interferons are involved in the recovery process. *(Reproduced, with permission, from Brooks GF et al.* Jawetz's Medical Microbiology, *22e. New York: McGraw-Hill, 2001.)*

123. The answer is b. *(Brooks, pp 420–423. Levinson, pp 250–254. Murray—2002, pp 513–515. Ryan, pp 532–535.)* Enteroviruses (polio-, Coxsackie-, and echoviruses) are ingested in contaminated water and/or food. Their main replication occurs in the intestinal tract, and virus progeny may get into the blood. From blood, distant target organs (the CNS, for example) may become involved. Most enterovirus CNS infections are self-limited, but some may progress to a life-threatening stage. Mumps virus and coronaviruses are inhaled initially. Influenza does not replicate in lymphocytes and does not involve the CNS. HIV has not been shown to be transmitted by any type of insect vector.

124. The answer is e. (*Brooks, p 338. Levinson, p 228. Murray—2002, p 488. Ryan, p 472.*) With an acute case of primary infection by Epstein-Barr virus (EBV), such as infectious mononucleosis, IgM antibodies to VCA should be present. Antibodies to EBNA should be absent, as they usually appear two to three months after onset of illness. Culture is not clinically useful because it (1) requires freshly fractionated cord blood lymphocytes, (2) takes three to four weeks for completion, and (3) is reactive in the majority of seropositive patients.

125. The answer is a. (*Brooks, p 367. Levinson, pp 231–233. Murray—2002, p 468. Ryan, p 508.*) While the herpesviruses (HSV, CMV, VZV) are all well known for latency, adenovirus can also form a latent infection in the lymphoid tissue. In 50 to 80% of surgically removed tonsils or adenoids, adenovirus can be cultured. The virus has also been cultured from mesenteric lymph nodes, and, in rare cases, viral DNA has been detected in peripheral lymphocytes. Recurrent illness usually does not arise from these latent infections; however, activation can occur in the immunosuppressed.

126. The answer is b. (*Brooks, pp 461–463. Levinson, p 238. Murray—2002, pp 541–542. Ryan, p 501.*) The symptoms described are consistent with influenza virus infection. The titers of antibody on November 6 and 30 show low levels of antibody against swine influenza, but indicate at least a measurable amount. The 160 titer on December 20 reflects a definitive diagnostic rise in antibody against swine influenza (>1:4 rise between acute and convalescent sera).

The previous titers (10 or 1:10) most likely represent cross-reacting antibodies from a non–swine influenza virus hemagglutinin or neuraminidase enzymes, which could account for cross-reacting antibodies.

127. The answer is c. (*Brooks, p 387. Levinson, p 228. Murray—2002, p 490. Ryan, p 572.*) Atypical lymphocytes are the hematologic hallmark of infectious mononucleosis with 90% or more of the circulating lymphocytes being atypical in some cases. These abnormal lymphocytes are not pathognomonic for infectious mononucleosis. They are also seen in other diseases, including cytomegalovirus infection, viral hepatitis, toxoplasmosis, rubella, mumps, and roseola.

128. The answer is a. (*Brooks, pp 451–452. Levinson, pp 270–271. Murray—2002, p 564. Ryan, p 592.*) Dengue (breakbone fever) is caused by a group B togavirus that is transmitted by mosquitoes. The clinical syndrome usually consists of a mild systemic disease characterized by severe joint and muscle pain, headache, fever, lymphadenopathy, and a maculopapular rash. Hemorrhagic dengue, a more severe syndrome, may be prominent during some epidemics; shock and, occasionally, death result.

129. The answer is e. (*Brooks, p 415. Levinson, pp 263–264. Murray—2002, pp 601–603. Ryan, pp 551–552.*) HCV is a positive-stranded RNA virus, classified as a Flavivirus. About half of HCV patients develop chronic hepatitis. A large number of infections appear among IV drug abusers. About 90% of the cases of transfusion-associated hepatitis are thought to be caused by HCV.

130–133. The answers are 130-c, 131-e, 132-b, 133-a. (*Brooks, p 412. Levinson, pp 261–262. Murray—2002, pp 600–601. Ryan, pp 548–549.*) Advances in the serodiagnosis of viral hepatitis have been dramatic, and the findings of specific viral antigens have led to further elucidation of the course of infections. The "Australia antigen," discovered in 1960, was first renamed hepatitis-associated antigen (HAA) and then, finally, hepatitis B surface antigen (HBsAg). It appears in the blood early after infection, before onset of acute illness, and persists through early convalescence. HBsAg usually disappears within four to six months after the start of clinical illness, except in the case of chronic carriers.

Hepatitis B 37 antigen (HBeAg) appears during the early acute phase and disappears before HBsAg is gone, although it may persist in the chronic carrier. Persons who are HBeAg-positive have higher titers of HBV and therefore are at a higher risk of transmitting the disease. HBeAg has a high correlation with DNA polymerase activity.

The hepatitis B core antigen (HBcAg) is found within the nuclei of infected hepatocytes and not generally in the peripheral circulation except as an integral component of the Dane particle. The antibody to this antigen, anti-HBc, is present at the beginning of clinical illness. As long as there is ongoing HBV replication, there will be high titers of anti-HBc. During the early convalescent phase of an HBV infection, anti-HBc may be the only detectable serologic marker (window phase) if HBsAg is negative and anti-HBsAg has not appeared.

134–138. The answers are 134-a, 135-b, 136-d, 137-c, 138-e. *(Brooks, pp 382–386, 478–480, 496, 429–431. Levinson, pp 226–227, 241–242, 242–244, 245–247, 254–255. Murray—2002, pp 493, 521, 530–531, 532–533, 551–552. Ryan, pp 510, 503–505, 513–514, 567–568, 598.)* Cytomegalovirus causes cytomegalic inclusion disease (CID), especially congenital abnormalities, in neonates. Malformations include microencephaly. Seizures, deafness, jaundice, and purpura can also occur. CID is also one of the leading causes of mental retardation in the United States. Orchitis, a complication of mumps virus infection in postpubertal males, can cause sterility if bilateral. Respiratory syncytial virus (RSV) is the leading cause of pneumonia and bronchiolitis in infants. Viremia does not occur and treatment in several ill infants is aerosolized ribavirin. The rabies virus is transmitted by the bite of a rabid animal. It almost always causes a fatal encephalitis if untreated. Postexposure treatment includes use of a killed vaccine and human rabies globulin (HIG). Rhinoviruses are the most prominent cause of the common cold. Many serotypes exist, which may account for their ability to cause frequent disease.

139–143. The answers are 139-c, 140-b, 141-d, 142-a, 143-d. *(Brooks, pp 349, 416–417, 468–469, 484. Levinson, pp 207–209, 238–239, 241, 258–259, 261–262. Murray—2002, pp 60, 149, 151–152, 483. Ryan, pp 502–503, 518, 544, 549, 561–562.)* The original vaccine for hepatitis B was prepared by purifying hepatitis B surface antigen (HBsAg) from healthy HBsAg-positive carriers and treating it with viral-inactivating agents. The second-generation vaccine for hepatitis B is produced by recombinant DNA in yeast cells containing a plasmid into which the gene for HBsAg has been incorporated.

Influenza usually occurs in successive waves of infection with peak incidences during the winter months. If only minor antigenic drift is expected for the next influenza season, then the most recent strains of A and B viruses representative of the main antigens are included in the vaccine. Influenza vaccine consists of killed viruses.

Live attenuated measles virus vaccine effectively prevents measles. Protection is provided if given before or within two days of exposure. Vaccination confers immunity for at least 15 years.

Acyclovir is an analogue of guanosine or deoxyguanosine that strongly inhibits herpes simplex virus (HSV) but has little effect on other DNA viruses. When employed for the treatment of primary genital infection by HSV, both oral and intravenous formulations have reduced viral shedding and shortened the duration of symptoms.

The vaccine for hepatitis A virus (HAV) is prepared from virus grown in culture and inactivated with formalin. Passive immunization with immune serum globulin confers passive protection in 90% of those exposed when given within one to two weeks after exposure.

144–148. The answers are 144-e, 145-a, 146-c, 147-d, 148-c. *(Brooks, pp 366–369, 378–379, 384, 436–438, 512–513. Levinson, pp 225–226, 231–233. Murray—2002, pp 458, 467, 484, 494–495, 548. Ryan, pp 509–510, 564–565, 568, 579, 619.)* Varicella-zoster virus is a herpesvirus. Chickenpox is a highly contagious disease of childhood that occurs in the late winter and early spring. It is characterized by a generalized vesicular eruption with relatively insignificant systemic manifestations.

Adenovirus has been associated with adult respiratory disease among newly enlisted military troops. Crowded conditions and strenuous exercise may account for the severe infections seen in this otherwise healthy group.

Papillomavirus is one of two members of the family Papovaviridae, which includes viruses that produce human warts. These viruses are host-specific and produce benign epithelial tumors that vary in location and clinical appearance. The warts usually occur in children and young adults and are limited to the skin and mucous membranes.

Rotavirus is worldwide in distribution and has been implicated as the major etiologic agent of infantile gastroenteritis. Infection with this virus varies in its clinical presentation from asymptomatic infection to a relatively mild diarrhea to a severe and sometimes fatal dehydration. The exact mode of transmission of this infectious agent is not known. Because of severe side effects, the rotavirus vaccine has been recalled and is temporarily unavailable.

Infectious mononucleosis caused by cytomegalovirus (CMV) is clinically difficult to distinguish from that caused by Epstein-Barr virus. Lymphocytosis is usually present, with an abundance of atypical lymphocytes. CMV-induced mononucleosis should be considered in any case of mononucleosis that is heterophil-negative and in patients with fever of unknown origin.

149–153. The answers are 149-b, 150-b, 151-c, 152-a, 153-a. (*Brooks, pp 386–388, 481–484, 584. Levinson, pp 227–229, 323–324. Murray—2002, pp 487–492, 525–528, 718–720. Ryan, pp 515–518, 569–572, 724.*) Epstein-Barr virus (EBV) is a herpesvirus that causes a number of syndromes; the most common is infectious mononucleosis. It is a ubiquitous enveloped DNA virus. Only one serotype of EBV has been recognized, although molecular methods have reorganized a number of genotypes of EBV.

Complement fixation antibody measurements against viruses may be a useful diagnostic tool if two serum samples are collected from the patient. The acute serum is collected as early in the illness as possible, and the convalescent serum is collected 7 to 10 days later. Both are included in the same test run against measles CF antigen. A positive diagnostic test occurs in the antibody titer when the convalescent serum is fourfold or greater than the acute sample. The sera are diluted in a twofold manner (1:2, 1:4, 1:8, etc.) for quantitation. The measures given above (40 and 80) are considered essentially the same level of antibodies in both samples. This patient must have had measles in the past and has the same amount of antibody in both serum samples.

Infectious mononucleosis is an acute disease most commonly seen in younger people. It is characterized by a proliferation of lymphocytes, lymph node enlargement, pharyngitis, fatigue, and fever. Infection in young children is usually either asymptomatic or characteristic of an acute upper respiratory infection. Diagnosis is usually made by a positive heterophil test. Heterophil antibodies are those that occur in one species (human) and react with antigens of a different species. The heterophil test may be insensitive (30 to 60%) in children. Definitive diagnosis is made by detection of antibodies to EBV components. EBV causes a variety of other syndromes including Burkitt's lymphoma, the most common childhood cancer in Africa, and nasopharyngeal carcinoma, commonly seen in China. Similar mononucleosis-like diseases are caused by cytomegalovirus (CMV) and *Toxoplasma gondii,* a parasite. CMV causes fewer than 10% of infectious mononucleosis-like diseases. CMV "mono" is primarily characterized by fatigue. Congenital infection with CMV almost always causes serious sequelae, such as retardation and hearing loss. *T. gondii* also causes a variety of clinical problems, among them encephalitis in AIDS patients and food poisoning from the ingestion of raw meat. Although CMV and *T. gondii* are relatively rare causes of infectious mononucleosis, they must be ruled out, particularly when EBV tests are nonreactive.

154–158. The answers are 154-b, 155-a, 156-b, 157-d, 158-d. (*Brooks, pp 615–617. Murray—2002, p 451. Ryan, p 231.*) The diagnosis of a viral infection is made easier by the creation of a greater number of diagnostic virology laboratories during the past few decades. In order for viral diagnosis to be successful, the most appropriate specimen must be collected for the disease in question.

Human papillomavirus (HPV) is often detected microscopically in cervical biopsies. Alternatively, there are methods to detect HPV DNA in such tissues as well as to serotype the virus. Evidence suggests that some HPV serotypes are more likely than others to cause cervical cancer.

Many viruses have a viremic phase, but only a few, such as CMV, persist after the patient becomes symptomatic. CMV can be isolated from lymphocytes and polymorphonuclear leukocytes. This usually requires special separation procedures, particularly in those compromised patients who may be neutropenic.

Enteroviruses such as echoviruses and coxsackieviruses are the predominant cause of aseptic viral meningitis. While enterovirus infections are often diagnosed by specific antibody response, it is possible to isolate the virus from CSF. Herpes simplex virus (HSV) can also be isolated from CSF in cases of herpes encephalitis or meningitis.

VZV and HSV are most often recovered from skin lesions, although varicella IgM antibody detection may be the most rapid way to diagnose acute VZV infection. Detection and identification of these viruses is essential because of the availability of antiviral agents such as acyclovir. Other viruses, such as enteroviruses and paramyxoviruses, cause skin lesions.

Many viruses can be isolated from feces. Of the viral groups in these questions, adenovirus 40/41 is the most common stool isolate. Norwalk agent and other caliciviruses may also be isolated or detected from stools, but usually only in specialized laboratories.

159–163. The answers are 159-c, 160-a, 161-e, 162-d, 163-b. (*Brooks, p 437. Howard, pp 833–836. Murray—2002, pp 612–614. Ryan, p 578.*) A number of viruses that cause gastroenteritis are now being recognized. The following table summarizes the characteristics of rotavirus, Norwalk virus, adenovirus, calicivirus, and astrovirus. (Table, p. 103.)

164–168. The answers are 164-a, 165-c, 166-b, 167-e, 168-d. (*Brooks, p 403. Levinson, pp 257–266. Murray—2002, p 592. Ryan, p 542.*) Hepatitis A virus (HAV) possesses a single-stranded linear RNA genome, while hepatitis B virus (HBV) contains a double-stranded DNA genome. Detection of anti-HAV IgM in a single serum specimen obtained in the acute or convalescent stage is the quickest and most reliable method to diagnose hepatitis A infection. This antibody is usually present at onset of symptoms and may persist three to six months. Demonstration of hepatitis B surface antigen (HBsAg) in serum is the most common method of diagnosing HBV infection. Other serologic markers helpful in characterizing infection with HBV include hepatitis B surface antibody (anti-HBs), anti-hepatitis B core (anti-HBc), anti-hepatitis B e antigen (anti-HBe), and hepatitis B e antigen (HBeAg). Several epidemiologic studies have demonstrated that immune serum globulin (ISG) can prevent clinical hepatitis A even when given up to 10 days after exposure. Similar studies have shown that ISG was able to decrease the incidence of hepatitis B infection in exposed persons. Purified, noninfectious HBsAg derived from healthy HBsAg carriers has been used as a vaccine for active immunization for HBV infection. Hepatitis C is a single-stranded RNA virus belonging to the family Flaviviridae. The viral reservoir is human. Recent retrospective "lookbacks" suggest that many people were infected with HCV before testing of the blood supply was initiated in the early 1990s. HCV is treatable with combinations of drugs. The genotype of the virus plays an important role in the determination of length of therapy. Hepatitis D virus is an incomplete or defective virus that requires HBsAg as a cofactor. Both co-infection and secondary delta infection exist, with secondary infection being the most serious. Hepatitis E virus is an RNA virus. Transmission is by the fecal-oral route, although maternal-fetal transmission has recently been described. Prognosis is usually favorable with rare cases of fulminant HEV reported.

169–172. The answers are 169-a, 170-e, 171-b, 172-b. (*Brooks, pp 375–376. Levinson, pp 221–224. Murray—2002, pp 479–481. Ryan pp*

	Norwalk and Norwalk-like Viruses	Rotavirus	Others		
			Adenovirus	Calicivirus	Astrovirus
Size (nm) diameter	27–35	70	70–90	35–39	28–30
Nucleic acid	RNA (single-stranded)	RNA (double-stranded)	DNA	RNA	RNA
Minimum number of serotypes	3	4 (3 groups, A, B, C)	2	3–5	5
Seasonality (temperate climate)	Winter	Winter	All seasons	—	—
Epidemicity	Epidemic	Sporadic, epidemic	Sporadic	Epidemic	Sporadic
Age with clinical disease	≥6 yr	6–24 mo most common	≤2 yr	≤2 yr	≤7 yr
Transmission	Fecal-oral, water, food	Fecal-oral, water, food	Fecal-oral	Fecal-oral	Fecal-oral

Source: Adapted, with permission, from Howard BJ, Keiser JF, Smith TF, Weissfeld AS, Tilton RC: *Clinical and Pathogenic Microbiology*, 2/e, St. Louis, Mosby, 1993.

559–561.) Human papillomaviruses (HPV) are the causative agents of cutaneous warts as well as proliferative squamous lesions of mucosal surfaces. Although most infections by human papillomavirus are benign, some undergo malignant transformation into in situ and invasive squamous cell carcinoma. Both HPV and polyomavirus have icosahedral capsids and DNA genomes. JC virus, a polyomavirus, was first isolated from the diseased brain of a patient with Hodgkin's lymphoma who was dying of progressive multifocal leukoencephalopathy (PML). This demyelinating disease occurs usually in immunosuppressed persons and is the result of oligodendrocyte infection by JC virus. JC virus has also been isolated from the urine of patients suffering from demyelinating disease. Cryotherapy and laser treatment are the most popular therapies for warts, although surgery may be indicated in some cases. At the present time, there is no effective antiviral therapy for treatment of infection with polyomavirus or HPV. West Nile virus (WNV) is an arbovirus. Although prevalent in Europe, Africa, and the Middle East, it was not seen in the United States until the summer of 1999. It is transmitted by mosquitoes and birds, especially crows; these animals are a reservoir. WNV causes a rather mild encephalitis in humans, the exception being older patients or those who may be immunocompromised.

Primary HSV-1 infections are usually asymptomatic. Symptomatic disease occurs most frequently in small children (one to five years old). Buccal and gingival mucosa are most often involved, and lesions, if untreated, may last two to three weeks. Acyclovir treatment is effective therapy and should be started immediately. The classic location of latent HSV-1 infection is the trigeminal ganglia. Reactivation results in sporadic vesicular lesions and may also be treated with acyclovir. B cell activation would be unusual, and there appears to be no greater risk for cancer development than that seen in the general population.

173–177. The answers are 173-b, 174-c, 175-e, 176-d, 177-a. (Brooks, pp 459, 473. Levinson, pp 235–239. Murray—2002, pp 524, 539–540. Ryan, pp 499–511.) Orthomyxoviruses and paramyxoviruses are RNA viruses that contain a single-stranded RNA genome. The influenza viruses belong to the orthomyxoviruses. They cause acute respiratory tract infections that usually occur in epidemics. Isolated strains of influenza virus are named after the virus type (influenza A, B, or C) as well as the host and location of initial isolation, the year of isolation, and the antigenic designation of the hemagglutinin and neuraminidase. Both the hemagglutinin and neuraminidase are glycoproteins under separate genetic control, and because of this they can and do vary independently. The changes in these antigens are responsible for the antigenic drift characteristic of these viruses. The paramyxoviruses include several important human pathogens (mumps virus, measles virus, respiratory syncytial virus, and parainfluenza virus). Both paramyxoviruses and orthomyxoviruses possess an RNA-dependent RNA polymerase that is a structural component of the virion and produces the initial RNA. Respiratory syncytial viruses (RSVs) are not related to the paramyxoviruses. They are 150-nm single-stranded RNA viruses. There are two antigen groups, A and B, which play no role in diagnosis and treatment. While the overall mortality rate is 0.5%, for at-risk groups mortality may be 25 to 35% if untreated. Some parainfluenza virus infections (type 3) may be indistinguishable from RSV, but most parainfluenza infections produce a laryngotracheobronchitis known as croup.

Bacteriology

Questions

DIRECTIONS: Each question below contains four or more suggested responses. Select the **one best** response to each question.

178. A patient with a peptic ulcer was admitted to the hospital and a gastric biopsy was performed. The tissue was cultured on chocolate agar incubated in a microaerophilic environment at 37°C for five to seven days. At five days of incubation, colonies appeared on the plate and curved, gram-negative rods, oxidase-positive, were observed. Which of the following is the most likely identity of this organism?

a. *Campylobacter fetus*
b. *Campylobacter jejuni*
c. *Haemophilus influenzae*
d. *Helicobacter pylori*
e. *Vibrio parahaemolyticus*

179. An inhibitor was designed to block a biologic function in *H. influenzae*. If the goal of the experiment was to reduce the virulence of *H. influenzae,* the most likely target would be which of the following?

a. Capsule formation
b. Endotoxin assembly
c. Exotoxin liberator
d. Flagella synthesis
e. IgA protease synthesis

180. An experimental compound is discovered that prevents the activation of adenylate cyclase and the resulting increase in cyclic AMP. The toxic effects of which of the following bacteria might be prevented with the use of this experimental compound?

a. *Brucella abortus*
b. *Corynebacterium diphtheriae*
c. *Listeria monocytogenes*
d. *Pseudomonas aeruginosa*
e. *Vibrio cholerae*

181. A single, 30-year-old woman presented to her physician with vaginitis. She complained of a slightly increased, malodorous discharge that was gray-white in color, thin, and homogenous. Clue cells were discovered when the discharge was examined microscopically. Which organism listed below was the most likely cause of her infection?

a. *Candida albicans*
b. *Trichomonas vaginalis*
c. *Escherichia coli*
d. *Gardnerella vaginalis*
e. *Staphylococcus aureus*

182. A 12-year-old girl was playing soccer when she began to limp. She has pain in her right leg and upper right thigh. Her temperature is 102°F. X-ray of the femur reveals that the periosteum is eroded, suggestive of osteomyelitis. Blood culture yields gram-positive bacteria. Which of the following is the most likely etiologic agent?

a. *L. monocytogenes*
b. *Salmonella enteritidis*
c. *Staphylococcus saprophyticus*
d. *S. aureus*
e. *Streptococcus pneumoniae*

183. A scraping from a painful, inflamed wound is found to contain numerous gram-negative bacteria. Upon questioning, the feverish patient states that he was bitten by a cat while trying to rescue it from a storm drain earlier in the day. Given these observations, which of the following organisms is the most likely cause of infection?

a. *Aeromonas* species
b. *C. jejuni*
c. *Pasteurella multocida*
d. *P. aeruginosa*
e. *Yersinia enterocolitica*

Item 184–186

A 21-year-old college student complained of malaise, low-grade fever, and a harsh cough, but not of muscle aches and pains. An x-ray revealed a diffuse interstitial pneumonia in the left lobes of the lung. The white blood cell (WBC) count was normal. The student had been ill for a week.

184. Based on the information given, which of the following is the most likely diagnosis?

a. Influenza
b. Legionellosis
c. Mycoplasma pneumonia
d. Pneumococcal pneumonia
e. Staphylococcal pneumonia

185. Based on the information given, which of the following laboratory tests would most rapidly assist you in making the diagnosis?

a. Cold agglutinins
b. Complement fixation (CF) test
c. Culture of sputum
d. Gram stain of sputum
e. Viral culture

186. The following laboratory data were available within two days: cold agglutinins—negative; complement fixation (*Mycoplasma pneumoniae*)—1:64; viral culture—pending, but negative to date; bacterial culture of sputum on blood agar and MacConkey's agar—normal oral flora. In order to confirm the diagnosis, which of the following procedures could be ordered to achieve a specific and sensitive diagnosis?

a. A DNA probe to the 16S ribosomal RNA of an organism lacking a cell wall
b. Another viral culture in one week
c. A repeat CF test in five days
d. A repeat cold agglutinin test
e. Culture of the sputum on charcoal yeast extract

187. Pathogenic mechanisms involved in tuberculosis can be primarily attributed to which of the following?

a. Cell-mediated hypersensitivity
b. Clogging of alveoli by large numbers of acid-fast mycobacteria
c. Humoral immunity
d. Specific cell adhesion sites
e. Toxin production by the mycobacteria

188. The class of antibiotics known as the quinolones is bactericidal. Which of the following characterizes their mode of action on growing bacteria?

a. Inactivation of penicillin-binding protein II
b. Inhibition of β-lactamase
c. Inhibition of DNA gyrase
d. Inhibition of reverse transcriptase
e. Prevention of the cross-linking of glycine

189. Vancomycin-indeterminate *S. aureus* (VISA) has recently been reported in the United States. Which one of the statements concerning VISA is the most correct?

a. Patients with VISA isolates need not be isolated
b. Minimum inhibitory concentration (MIC) for vancomycin is at least 1.0 mcg/mL
c. VISAs have emerged because of the extended use of vancomycin for methicillin-resistant *S. aureus* (MRSAs)
d. VISA isolates are infrequent, so surveillance at the present time is not warranted
e. VISA isolates are usually methicillin susceptible (MRSA)

190. A sputum sample was brought to the laboratory for analysis. Gram stain revealed the following: rare epithelial cells, 8 to 10 polymorphonuclear leukocytes per high-power field, and pleomorphic gram-negative rods. As a laboratory consultant, which of the following interpretations should you make?

a. The appearance of the sputum is suggestive of *H. influenzae*
b. The patient has pneumococcal pneumonia
c. The patient has Vincent's disease
d. The sputum specimen is too contaminated by saliva to be useful
e. There is no evidence of an inflammatory response

191. A 25-year-old medical student presented with a burst appendix. A peritoneal infection developed, despite prompt removal of the organ and extensive flushing of the peritoneal cavity. An isolate from a pus culture was a gram-negative rod identified as *Bacteroides fragilis.* Anaerobic infection with *B. fragilis* is characterized by which one of the following?

a. A black exudate in the wound
b. A foul-smelling discharge
c. A heme-pigmented colony formation
d. An exquisite susceptibility to penicillin
e. Severe neurologic symptoms

192. Several days after an unprotected sexual encounter, a healthy 21-year-old male develops pain and pus on urination. A Gram stain reveals gram-negative diplococci. Which of the following structures is most responsible for adherence of the offending microbe to the urethral mucosa?

a. Capsule
b. Fimbriae
c. Flagella
d. The F pili
e. The peptidoglycan
f. The LPS

193. A 4-week-old newborn developed meningitis. Short, gram-positive rods were isolated and identified as *Listeria* organisms. The mother had eaten unpasteurized cheese from Mexico during the pregnancy and recalled having a flulike illness. *L. monocytogenes* causes a variety of diseases, including food poisoning. Which of the following best describes these microorganisms?

a. Flagella are produced both at room temperature and at 37°C
b. *Listeria* are facultative intracellular pathogens
c. *Listeria* cannot be cultivated on artificial media
d. Once infected, the immune system cannot destroy *Listeria*
e. There is no relationship between *Listeria* serovars and human infection

Questions 194–197

194. A 30-year-old male patient was seen by the emergency service and reported a two-week history of a penile ulcer. He noted that this ulcer did not hurt. Which one of the following conclusions/actions is most valid?

a. Draw blood for a herpes antibody test
b. Even if treated, the lesion will remain for months
c. Failure to treat the patient will have no untoward effect, as this is a self-limiting infection
d. Perform a dark-field examination of the lesion
e. Prescribe acyclovir for primary genital herpes

195. The laboratory reports that the Venereal Disease Research Laboratory (VDRL) test performed on the patient in question 194 is reactive at a dilution of 1:4 (4 dils). The patient also reports to you that he has recently been diagnosed with hepatitis A. Which one of the following actions would be most appropriate?

a. Order a confirmatory test such as the fluorescent treponemal antibody (FTA) test
b. Order a rapid plasma reagin (RPR) test
c. Perform a spinal tap to rule out CNS syphilis
d. Repeat the VDRL test
e. Report this patient to the health department, as he has syphilis

196. In the same patient, which one of the following test combinations for syphilis is most appropriate?

a. FTA-Abs (IgG)/FTA-Abs (IgM)
b. RPR/culture of the lesion
c. RPR/FTA-Abs
d. *Treponema pallidum* hemagglutination (TPHA)/microhemagglutination—*T. pallidum* (MHTP) tests
e. VDRL/RPR

197. Assume that the patient absolutely denied any contact, sexual or otherwise, with a person who had syphilis. Assume also that both the RPR and the FTA-Abs were positive on this patient. Which one of the following tests could be used to show that this patient probably does not have syphilis?

a. Frei test
b. MHTP test
c. Quantitative RPR
d. *T. pallidum* immobilization (TPI) test
e. VDRL

198. A 55-year-old man who is being treated for adenocarcinoma of the lung is admitted to a hospital because of a temperature of 38.9°C (102°F), chest pain, and a dry cough. Sputum is collected. Gram stain of the sputum is unremarkable, and culture reveals many small, gram-negative rods able to grow only on a charcoal yeast extract agar. This organism most likely is which of the following?

a. *Chlamydia trachomatis*
b. *Klebsiella pneumoniae*
c. *Legionella pneumophila*
d. *M. pneumoniae*
e. *S. aureus*

199. A patient was hospitalized after an automobile accident. The wounds became infected and the patient was treated with tobramycin, carbenicillin, and clindamycin. Five days after antibiotic therapy was initiated, the patient developed severe diarrhea and pseudomembranous enterocolitis. Antibiotic-associated diarrhea and the more serious pseudomembranous enterocolitis can be caused by which of the following organisms?

a. *B. fragilis*
b. *Clostridium difficile*
c. *Clostridium perfringens*
d. *Clostridium sordellii*
e. *S. aureus*

200. A premature neonate suffers pneumonia and sepsis. Sputum culture on blood agar plate yields pin-pointed β-hemolytic colonies. Which of the following is a simple test to determine whether the organism is *Streptococcus agalactiae* or *L. monocytogenes* (these two organisms are important neonatal pathogens)?

a. Bacitracin sensitivity test
b. Catalase test
c. Coagulase test
d. Polymerase chain reaction
e. Sugar fermentation test

201. A 2-year-old child has a high fever and is irritable. He has a stiff neck. Gram stain smear of spinal fluid reveals gram-negative, small pleomorphic coccobacillary organisms. What is the most appropriate procedure to follow in order to reach an etiological diagnosis?

a. Culture the spinal fluid in chocolate agar and identify the organism by growth factors
b. Culture the spinal fluid in mannitol-salt agar
c. Perform a catalase test of the isolated organism
d. Perform a coagulase test with the isolate
e. Perform a latex agglutination test to detect the specific antibody in the spinal fluid

202. A patient complained to his dentist about a draining lesion in his mouth. A Gram stain of the pus showed a few gram-positive cocci, leukocytes, and many-branched gram-positive rods. Which of the following is the most likely cause of the disease?

a. *Actinomyces israelii*
b. *Actinomyces viscosus*
c. *C. diphtheriae*
d. *Propionibacterium acnes*
e. *S. aureus*

Questions 203–205

203. A female infant was born prematurely after rupture of membranes and, within one day of birth, developed a fever and died. The pregnant mother had been cultured just prior to the birth of her child and her vaginal culture revealed group B streptococci (*S. agalactiae*). Which one of the tests shown in the following figure would provide the most rapid and useful information?

a. A
b. B
c. C
d. D

A.

C.

B.

D.

A. Direct Gram stain demonstrating *Streptococcus agalactiae* in CSF of infected neonate (μ1000). **B.** Blood agar plate demonstrating diffuse β-hemolysis due to group B streptococci from CSF. **C.** Brain at autopsy demonstrating acute hemorrhagic response to *S. agalactiae*. **D.** Brain section with blood vessel occluded by group B streptococci.

204. Group B streptococcus sepsis in an infant is preventable. Which one of the following procedures is most likely to reduce the incidence of group B streptococcal disease?

a. Identification of possible high-risk births
b. Intrapartum antibiotic treatment
c. Screening of pregnant females at the first office visit, usually during the first trimester
d. Screening of pregnant females in the last trimester
e. Use of a polysaccharide vaccine

205. There has been much speculation on the pathogenesis of group B streptococcal disease in the neonate. Which of the following is one of the most likely pathogenic mechanisms?

a. Complement C5a, a potent chemoattractant, activates PMNs
b. In the absence of a specific antibody, opsonization, phagocyte recognition, and killing do not proceed normally
c. The alternative complement pathway is activated
d. The streptococci are resistant to penicillin

206. A man who has a penile chancre appears in a hospital's emergency service. The VDRL test is negative. What is the most appropriate course of action for the physician in charge?

a. Perform dark-field microscopy for treponemes
b. Perform a Gram stain on the chancre fluid
c. Repeat the VDRL test in 10 days
d. Send the patient home untreated
e. Swab the chancre and culture on Thayer-Martin agar

207. A mentally depressed farmer complains of great weakness, a daily rise and fall in fever, and night sweats. Small gram-negative rods were isolated from blood cultures after two weeks' incubation. The organism that is most likely to be the etiologic agent is which of the following?

a. *Brucella melitensis*
b. *C. jejuni*
c. *Francisella tularensis*
d. *S. enteritidis*
e. *Serratia marcescens*

208. An outbreak occurred in a community where the water supply was contaminated. Multiple patients experienced nausea and vomiting, as well as profuse diarrhea with abdominal cramps. Stools were described as "rice water." Curved, gram-negative rods were isolated on this sulfate-citrate-bile-sucrose agar. In the treatment of patients who have cholera, the use of a drug that inhibits adenyl cyclase would be expected to have which of the following characteristics?

a. Block the action of cholera toxin
b. Eradicate the organism
c. Increase fluid secretion
d. Kill the patient immediately
e. Reduce intestinal motility

209. A box of ham sandwiches with mayonnaise, prepared by a person with a boil on his neck, was left out of the refrigerator for the on-call interns. Three doctors became violently ill approximately two hours after eating the sandwiches. The most likely cause is which of the following?

a. *C. perfringens* toxin
b. Coagulase from *S. aureus* in the ham
c. Penicillinase given to inactivate penicillin in the pork
d. *S. aureus* enterotoxin
e. *S. aureus* leukocidin

210. *S. aureus* causes a wide variety of infections, ranging from wound infection to pneumonia. Which of the following often complicates treatment of *S. aureus* infection with penicillin?

a. Allergic reaction caused by staphylococcal protein
b. Inability of penicillin to penetrate the membrane of *S. aureus*
c. Lack of penicillin binding sites on *S. aureus*
d. Production of penicillin acetylase by *S. aureus*
e. Production of penicillinase by *S. aureus*

211. Two of three family members had dinner at a local restaurant and within 48 hours, experienced double vision, difficulty in swallowing and speaking, and breathing problems. These symptoms are consistent with which of the following?

a. Activation of cyclic AMP
b. Endotoxin shock
c. Ingestion of a neurotoxin
d. Invasion of the gut epithelium by an organism
e. Secretion of an enterotoxin

212. Several *Neisseria* species are a part of the normal flora (commensals) of the human upper respiratory tract. Which of the following statements accurately describes the significance of these bacteria?

a. As a part of the normal flora, Neisseriae provide a natural immunity in local host defense
b. As a part of the respiratory flora, they are the most common cause of acute bronchitis and pneumonia
c. Commensal bacteria stimulate a cell-mediated immunity (CMI)
d. Commensal Neisseriae in the upper respiratory tract impede phagocytosis by means of lipoteichoic acid
e. Normal flora such as nonpathogenic Neisseriae provide effective nonspecific B-cell-mediated humoral immunity

213. A family routinely consumed unpasteurized milk, claiming "better taste." Several members experienced a sudden onset of crampy abdominal pain, fever, and a bloody, profane diarrhea. *C. jejuni* was isolated and identified from all patients. The treatment of choice for this type of enterocolitis is which of the following?

a. Ampicillin
b. *Campylobacter* antitoxin
c. Ciprofloxacin
d. Erythromycin
e. Pepto-Bismol

214. A hyperemic edema of the larynx and epiglottis that rapidly leads to respiratory obstruction in young children is most likely to be caused by which of the following organisms?

a. *Haemophilus hemolyticus*
b. *H. influenzae*
c. *K. pneumoniae*
d. *M. pneumoniae*
e. *Neisseria meningitidis*

Item 215–217

A 70-year-old female patient was readmitted to a local hospital with fever and chills following cardiac surgery at a major teaching institution. Blood cultures were taken and a gram-positive coccus grew from the blood cultures within 24 hours. Initial tests indicated that this isolate was resistant to penicillin.

215. Which of the following is the most likely identification?

a. Enterococcus
b. Group A streptococcus
c. Group B streptococcus
d. *Neisseria* species
e. *S. pneumoniae*

216. Further testing revealed that the isolate possessed the group D antigen, was not β-lactamase-positive, but was resistant to vancomycin. Which of the following is the most likely identification of this isolate?

a. *Enterococcus cassiflavus*
b. *Enterococcus durans*
c. *Enterococcus faecalis*
d. *Enterococcus faecium*
e. *S. pneumoniae*

217. Which of the following is the treatment of choice for the isolate in question 215?

a. Ciprofloxacin
b. Gentamicin
c. Gentamicin and ampicillin
d. Rifampin
e. No available treatment

218. Acute hematogenous osteomyelitis is often diagnosed by isolation of the organism from the blood and is caused most often by which of the following organisms?

a. *E. coli*
b. *Proteus mirabilis*
c. *S. aureus*
d. *Staphylococcus epidermidis*
e. *Streptococcus faecalis*

219. Diphtheria toxin is produced only by those strains of *C. diphtheriae* that have which of the following characteristics?

a. Encapsulated
b. Glucose fermenters
c. Lysogenic for β-prophage
d. Of the mitis strain
e. Sucrose fermenters

Item 220–222

A 28-year-old menstruating woman appeared in the emergency room with the following signs and symptoms: fever, 104°F (40°C); WBC, 16,000/μL; blood pressure, 90/65 mmHg; a scarlatiniform rash on her trunk, palms, and soles; extreme fatigue; vomiting; and diarrhea.

220. The patient described in this case most likely has which of the following?

a. Chickenpox
b. Guillain-Barré syndrome
c. Scalded skin syndrome
d. Staphylococcal food poisoning
e. Toxic shock syndrome

221. Culture of the menstrual fluid in the case cited would most likely reveal a predominance of which of the following?

a. *C. difficile*
b. *C. perfringens*
c. *G. vaginalis*
d. *S. aureus*
e. *S. epidermidis*

222. The most characteristic finding not yet revealed in the case just presented would be which of the following?

a. A meal of chicken in a fast-food restaurant
b. A retained tampon
c. Heavy menstrual flow
d. Recent exposure to rubella
e. Travel to Vermont

Item 223–224

A new latex agglutination (LA) reagent for *H. influenzae* polysaccharide antigen in cerebrospinal fluid was evaluated. Results were compared with the isolation of *H. influenzae* from the CSF. Results were as follows:

LA POS, CULT POS: 25
LA POS, CULT NEG: 5
LA NEG, CULT POS: 5
LA NEG, CULT NEG: 95

223. Which of the following best indicates the sensitivity of LA?

a. 0%
b. 30%
c. 85%
d. 95%
e. 100%

224. Which of the following best indicates the specificity of LA?

a. 0%
b. 30%
c. 80%
d. 95%
e. 100%

225. A severely burned firefighter develops a rapidly disseminating bacterial infection while hospitalized. "Green pus" is noted in the burned tissue, and cultures of both the tissue and blood yield small, oxidase-positive, gram-negative rods. Which of the following statements most accurately conveys information about this organism?

a. Endotoxin is the only virulence factor known to be produced by these bacteria
b. Humans are the only known reservoir hosts for these bacteria
c. The bacteria are difficult to culture because they have numerous growth requirements
d. These are among the most antibiotic resistant of all clinically relevant bacteria
e. These highly motile bacteria can "swarm" over the surface of culture media

226. Which of the following pairs of organisms can be routinely responsible for food poisoning?

a. *Clostridium botulinum* and *Bacillus anthracis*
b. *C. difficile* and *C. botulinum*
c. *C. perfringens* and *Bacillus cereus*
d. *Clostridium tetani* and *B. anthracis*
e. *C. tetani* and *B. cereus*

227. Methicillin-resistant *S. aureus* (MRSA) was isolated from seven patients in a 14-bed intensive care unit. All patients were isolated and the unit closed to any more admissions. Which one of the following reasons best explains these rigorous methods to control MRSA?

a. MRSA causes toxic shock syndrome
b. MRSA is inherently more virulent than other staphylococci
c. MRSA is resistant to penicillin
d. MRSA spreads more rapidly from patient to patient than antibiotic-susceptible staphylococci do
e. The alternative for treatment of MRSA is vancomycin, an expensive and potentially toxic antibiotic

228. A patient with AIDS returned from Haiti with acute diarrhea. The stool revealed an oval organism (8 to 9 μ in diameter) that was acid-fast and fluoresced blue under ultraviolet light. The most likely identification of this organism is which of the following?

a. *Cryptosporidium*
b. *Cyclospora*
c. *Enterocytozoon*
d. *Giardia*
e. *Prototheca*

229. A 2-year-old infant is brought to the emergency room with hemolytic uremic syndrome and thrombocytopenia. Which one of the following bacteria would most likely be isolated from a stool specimen?

a. *Aeromonas* species
b. *Enterobacter aerogenes*
c. *E. coli* 0157/H7
d. *S. enteriditis*
e. *Shigella flexneri*

230. *E. coli* causes disease by a variety of different methods. Which one of the following *E. coli* types is characterized by the presence of LT (heat-labile) and ST (heat-stable) proteins?

a. Enteroinvasive (EIEC)
b. Enterotoxigenic (ETEC)
c. Enterohemorrhagic (EHEC)
d. Enteropathogenic (EPEC)
e. Enterohemolytic (EHEEC)

231. *Yersinia pestis,* the causative agent of plague, is enzootic in the United States west of the one-hundredth meridian. Human plague can be bubonic or pneumonic. What is the primary epidemiologic difference between the two clinical forms of plague?

a. Age of the patient
b. Geographic location of the animal vector
c. Health of the animal vector
d. Route of infection
e. Season of the year

232. A 9-year-old child is brought to the emergency room with the chief complaint of enlarged, painful axillary lymph nodes. The resident physician also notes a small, inflamed, dime-sized lesion surrounding what appears to be a small scratch on the forearm. The lymph node is aspirated and some pus is sent to the laboratory for examination. A Warthin-Starry silver impregnation stain reveals many highly pleomorphic, rod-shaped bacteria. Which of the following is the most likely cause of this infection?

a. *Bartonella henselae*
b. *Brucella canis*
c. *Mycobacterium scrofulaceum*
d. *Y. enterocolitica*
e. *Y. pestis*

233. A sixth-grade boy returned from summer camp with several minor cuts and abrasions. Within a week, extensive cellulitis developed, and it was apparent that subcutaneous tissue was involved, requiring surgical intervention of nonviable tissue. Antibiotics were used aggressively. This necrotizing fasciitis is usually caused by which of the following?

a. *B. cereus*
b. *C. tetani*
c. Group A streptococci
d. *Micrococcus*
e. *S. aureus*

234. Which of the following is the most effective noninvasive test for the diagnosis of *Helicobacter*-associated gastric ulcers?

a. Culture of stomach contents for *H. pylori*
b. Detection of *H. pylori* antigen in stool
c. Growth of *H. pylori* from a stomach biopsy
d. Growth of *H. pylori* in the stool
e. IgM antibodies to *H. pylori*

235. The following test results were observed in a woman tested in November who reported being in the woods in Pennsylvania during the past summer, was bitten by a tick, and now has erythema migrans, a flattened red area near the bite with central clearing. She also has flulike illness with fever, myalgia, and headache: Lyme IgG antibody 1:1280; Lyme IgM antibody negative. Which one of the following courses of action is most appropriate?

a. Ask the patient if she has a severe headache
b. Ask the patient if she has had a urinary tract infection with *E. coli*
c. Consider treatment of the patient with an appropriate antibiotic such as tetracycline
d. Ignore the results because there is no Lyme disease in Pennsylvania
e. Order tests for syphilis (VDRL, FTA-Abs) because there are cross-reactions reported with *Borrelia burgdorferi*

236. *Mycobacterium avium* is a major opportunistic pathogen in AIDS patients. *M. avium* from AIDS patients can be best characterized by which one of the following statements?

a. Few isolates from AIDS patients are acid-fast
b. Most isolates from AIDS patients are sensitive to isoniazid and streptomycin
c. *M. avium* can be isolated from the blood of many AIDS patients
d. *M. avium* isolates from AIDS patients are of multiple serovars
e. The majority of *M. avium* isolates from AIDS patients are nonpigmented

237. Rheumatic fever (RF) is a disease seen in children and young adults. Which one of the following statements best typifies the disease?

a. It is a complication of group A streptococcal skin disease but usually not of pharyngitis
b. It is characterized by inflammatory lesions that may involve the heart, joints, subcutaneous tissues, and CNS
c. It is very common in developing countries but extremely rare and decreasing in incidence in the United States
d. Prophylaxis with benzathine penicillin is of little value
e. The pathogenesis is related to the similarity between a staphylococcal antigen and a human cardiac antigen

238. After extraction of a wisdom tooth, an 18-year-old male student was diagnosed as having subacute bacterial endocarditis. He has a congential heart disease that has been under control. Which of the following is the most likely organism causing his infection?

a. *S. aureus*
b. *S. epidermidis*
c. *S. pneumoniae*
d. *Streptococcus viridians*
e. *S. faecalis*

239. The patient is a 64-year-old sheepherder from the farming region of central California. He is rushed to the emergency room in anaphylactic shock. The history, as told by the ambulance medic, is that the man had been hit in the abdomen during a barroom brawl. Ultrasound reveals a large cyst mass in the liver. A cautious needle aspiration of the liver mass reveals "hydatid sand." Which of the following is the most likely agent involved?

a. *Ascaris*
b. *Clonorchis*
c. *Echinococcus*
d. *Fasciolopsis*
e. *Schistosoma*

240. If a quellung test was done on the following bacterial isolates, which one would you expect to be positive?

a. *C. diphtheriae*
b. *Enterobacter*
c. *Haemophilus parainfluenzae*
d. *Neisseria gonorrhoeae*
e. *S. pneumoniae*

241. A 2-year-old child was admitted to the hospital with acute meningitis. The Gram stain revealed gram-positive, short rods, and the mother indicated that the child had received "all" of the meningitis vaccinations. What is the most likely cause of the disease?

a. *H. influenzae*
b. *L. monocytogenes*
c. *N. meningitidis*, group A
d. *N. meningitidis*, group C
e. *S. pneumoniae*

Questions 242–245

242. Which of the following is the most common portal of entry for *C. tetani*, the cause of tetanus?

a. Gastrointestinal tract
b. Genital tract
c. Nasal tract
d. Respiratory tract
e. Skin

243. Which of the following is the most common way in which tuberculosis is acquired?

a. Gastrointestinal tract
b. Genital tract
c. Nasal tract
d. Respiratory tract
e. Skin

244. Shigellosis is common in travelers to developing countries. Infection is commonly acquired through which of the following routes?

a. Gastrointestinal tract
b. Genital tract
c. Nasal tract
d. Respiratory tract
e. Skin

245. A person who contracts gonorrhea is most likely to have acquired it via which of the following?

a. Gastrointestinal tract
b. Genital tract
c. Nasal tract
d. Respiratory tract
e. Skin

Questions 246–247

246. There are a variety of "unusual" bacteria that infect humans. While rare, disease caused by these microorganisms is serious and occasionally difficult to identify. Which of the following statements best characterizes *Moraxella (Branhamella) catarrhalis?*

a. A gram-negative, pleomorphic rod that can cause endocarditis
b. A gram-negative rod, fusiform-shaped, that is associated with periodontal disease but may cause sepsis
c. The causative agent of rat-bite fever
d. The causative agent of sinusitis, bronchitis, and pneumonia
e. The causative agent of trench fever

247. Which of the following statements best characterizes *Capnocytophaga?*

a. A gram-negative, pleomorphic rod that can cause endocarditis
b. A gram-negative rod, fusiform-shaped, that is associated with periodontal disease but may cause sepsis
c. The causative agent of rat-bite fever
d. The causative agent of sinusitis, bronchitis, and pneumonia
e. The causative agent of trench fever

248. The etiologic agent of Q fever is transmitted to man via which of the following methods?

a. Fecal contamination from flea deposits on the skin
b. Inhalation of infected aerosols from animal urine and feces
c. Lice feces scratched into the broken skin during the louse's blood feeding
d. Tick saliva during feeding on human blood
e. Urethral discharge from infected humans

Questions 249–250

249. An enterococcus (*E. faecium*) was isolated from a urine specimen (100,000 cfu/mL). Treatment of the patient with ampicillin and gentamicin failed. What is the most clinically appropriate action?

a. Consider vancomycin as an alternative drug
b. Determine if fluorescent microscopy is available for the diagnosis of actinomycosis
c. Do no further clinical workup
d. Suggest to the laboratory that low colony counts may reflect infection
e. Suggest a repeat antibiotic susceptibility test

250. A patient with symptoms of urinary tract infection had a culture taken, which grew 5×10^3 *E. coli*. The laboratory reported it as "insignificant." What is the most clinically appropriate action?

a. Consider vancomycin as an alternative drug
b. Determine if fluorescent microscopy is available for the diagnosis of actinomycosis
c. Do no further clinical workup
d. Suggest to the laboratory that low colony counts may reflect infection
e. Suggest a repeat antibiotic susceptibility test

251. A patient appeared in the emergency room with a submandibular mass. A smear was made of the drainage and a bewildering variety of bacteria were seen, including branched, gram-positive rods. What is the most clinically appropriate action?

a. Consider vancomycin as an alternative drug
b. Determine if fluorescent microscopy is available for the diagnosis of actinomycosis
c. Do no further clinical workup
d. Suggest to the laboratory that low colony counts may reflect infection
e. Suggest a repeat antibiotic susceptibility test

Questions 252–256

252. Which of the following is the antibiotic therapy of choice for legionellosis?

a. Ampicillin
b. Ceftriaxone
c. Erythromycin
d. Penicillin
e. Vancomycin

253. Which of the following is the antibiotic of choice for pneumococcal pneumonia?

a. Ampicillin
b. Ceftriaxone
c. Erythromycin
d. Penicillin
e. Vancomycin

254. Which of the following is the antibiotic of choice for Lyme disease?

a. Ampicillin
b. Ceftriaxone
c. Erythromycin
d. Penicillin
e. Vancomycin

255. Which of the following is the antibiotic of choice for streptococcal pharyngitis?

a. Ampicillin
b. Ceftriaxone
c. Erythromycin
d. Penicillin
e. Vancomycin

256. Which of the following is the therapy of choice for pseudomembranous enterocolitis?

a. Ampicillin
b. Ceftriaxone
c. Erythromycin
d. Penicillin
e. Vancomycin

Item 257–260

Although cholera, a *Vibrio* infection, has rarely been seen in the United States, there have been recent outbreaks of classic cholera associated with shellfish harvested from the Gulf of Mexico. Vibrios are shaped like curved rods, and infections more common than cholera may be caused by a variety of curved-rod bacteria.

257. Which of the following best describes *C. jejuni*?

a. Cause of gastroenteritis; reservoir in birds and mammals, optimal growth at 42°C
b. Human pathogen, halophilic, lactose-negative, sucrose-negative; causes gastrointestinal diseases primarily from ingestion of cooked seafood
c. Human pathogen, halophilic, lactose-positive; produces heat-labile, extracellular toxin
d. "String-test"-positive isolate; three serotypes—Ogawa (AB), Inaba (AC), Hikojima (ABC)
e. Urease-positive; cause of fetal distress in cattle

258. *V. cholerae,* the causative agent of cholera, is best described by which of the following statements?

a. Cause of gastroenteritis; reservoir in birds and mammals, optimal growth at 42°C
b. Human pathogen, halophilic, lactose-negative, sucrose-negative; causes gastrointestinal diseases primarily from ingestion of cooked seafood
c. Human pathogen, halophilic, lactose-positive; produces heat-labile, extracellular toxin
d. "String-test"-positive isolate; three serotypes—Ogawa (AB), Inaba (AC), Hikojima (ABC)
e. Urease-positive; cause of fetal distress in cattle

259. *V. parahaemolyticus,* first described in Japan, is best characterized by which of the following statements?

a. Cause of gastroenteritis; reservoir in birds and mammals, optimal growth at 42°C
b. Human pathogen, halophilic, lactose-negative, sucrose-negative; causes gastrointestinal diseases primarily from ingestion of cooked seafood
c. Human pathogen, halophilic, lactose-positive; produces heat-labile, extracellular toxin
d. "String-test"-positive isolate; three serotypes—Ogawa (AB), Inaba (AC), Hikojima (ABC)
e. Urease-positive; cause of fetal distress in cattle

260. *Vibrio vulnificus,* which can be found in the oceans and bays in temperate and tropical climates, is best characterized by which of the following statements?

a. Cause of gastroenteritis; reservoir in birds and mammals, optimal growth at 42°C
b. Human pathogen, halophilic, lactose-negative, sucrose-negative; causes gastrointestinal diseases primarily from ingestion of cooked seafood
c. Human pathogen, halophilic, lactose-positive; produces heat-labile, extracellular toxin
d. "String-test"-positive isolate; three serotypes—Ogawa (AB), Inaba (AC), Hikojima (ABC)
e. Urease-positive; cause of fetal distress in cattle

Item 261–264

Each of the following bacteria is a small, gram-negative rod. Some of them are fastidious and may be difficult to culture and identify. They have unique microbiological features, and each of them causes distinctive clinical disease.

261. *Y. enterocolitica,* formerly a *Pasteurella,* is best described by which of the following statements?

a. Commonly inhabits the canine respiratory tract and is an occasional pathogen for humans; strongly urease-positive
b. Manifests different biochemical and physiologic characteristics, depending on growth temperature, and causes a spectrum of human disease, most commonly mesenteric lymphadenitis
c. Pits agar, grows both in carbon dioxide and under anaerobic conditions, and is part of the normal oral cavity flora
d. Typically infects cattle, requires 5 to 10% carbon dioxide for growth, and is inhibited by the dye thionine
e. Typically is found in infected animal bites in humans and can cause hemorrhagic septicemia in animals

262. *B. abortus,* one of the three species causing brucellosis, a possible bioterrorism agent, is best described by which of the following statements?

a. Commonly inhabits the canine respiratory tract and is an occasional pathogen for humans; strongly urease-positive
b. Manifests different biochemical and physiologic characteristics, depending on growth temperature, and causes a spectrum of human disease, most commonly mesenteric lymphadenitis
c. Pits agar, grows both in carbon dioxide and under anaerobic conditions, and is part of the normal oral cavity flora
d. Typically infects cattle, requires 5 to 10% carbon dioxide for growth, and is inhibited by the dye thionine
e. Typically is found in infected animal bites in humans and can cause hemorrhagic septicemia in animals

263. *Bordetella bronchiseptica* could be confused with the agent of whooping cough. It is best described by which of the following statements?

a. Commonly inhabits the canine respiratory tract and is an occasional pathogen for humans; strongly urease-positive
b. Manifests different biochemical and physiologic characteristics, depending on growth temperature, and causes a spectrum of human disease, most commonly mesenteric lymphadenitis
c. Pits agar, grows both in carbon dioxide and under anaerobic conditions, and is part of the normal oral cavity flora
d. Typically infects cattle, requires 5 to 10% carbon dioxide for growth, and is inhibited by the dye thionine
e. Typically is found in infected animal bites in humans and can cause hemorrhagic septicemia in animals

264. *P. multocida* is a very common organism and is best described by which of the following statements?

a. Commonly inhabits the canine respiratory tract and is an occasional pathogen for humans; strongly urease-positive
b. Manifests different biochemical and physiologic characteristics, depending on growth temperature, and causes a spectrum of human disease, most commonly mesenteric lymphadenitis
c. Pits agar, grows both in carbon dioxide and under anaerobic conditions, and is part of the normal oral cavity flora
d. Typically infects cattle, requires 5 to 10% carbon dioxide for growth, and is inhibited by the dye thionine
e. Typically is found in infected animal bites in humans and can cause hemorrhagic septicemia in animals

Item 265–267

To isolate specific bacteria from clinical specimens, it is necessary to use a variety of artificial media, some of which are selective, others of which are nonselective.

265. *N. gonorrhoeae* is a fastidious pathogen found in sites often contaminated with normal flora. What is the best medium for isolation?

a. Löffler's medium
b. Löwenstein-Jensen medium
c. Sheep blood agar
d. Thayer-Martin agar
e. Thiosulfate citrate bile salts sucrose medium

266. *V. cholerae,* the causative agent of cholera, is best isolated using which one of the following?

a. Löffler's medium
b. Löwenstein-Jensen medium
c. Sheep blood agar
d. Thayer-Martin agar
e. Thiosulfate citrate bile salts sucrose medium

267. *Mycobacterium tuberculosis* can be found in the sputum of patients with tuberculosis. After digestion of the sputum, isolation is best accomplished using which one of the following?

a. Löffler's medium
b. Löwenstein-Jensen medium
c. Sheep blood agar
d. Thayer-Martin agar
e. Thiosulfate citrate bile salts sucrose medium

268. Antibiotic therapy is a critical step in the management of patients infected with each of the following microorganisms except for one. What is the exception?

a. *B. anthracis*
b. *C. botulinum*
c. *C. difficile*
d. *C. perfringens*
e. *C. tetani*

269. A 12-year-old boy has sudden onset of fever, headache, and stiff neck. Two days before, he swam in a lake that is believed to have been contaminated with dog excreta. Leptospirosis is suspected. What laboratory tests are most appropriate at this time to determine whether he has been infected with leptospira?

a. Agglutination test for leptospiral antigen
b. Counterimmunoelectrophoresis of urine sample
c. Gram stain of urine specimen
d. Spinal fluid for dark-field microscopy and culture in Fletcher's serum medium
e. Urine culture on EMB and Thayer-Martin agar

Item 270–273

In order to recognize abnormal bacteria, it is necessary to know which bacteria are predominant normal flora of certain body sites.

270. Which of the following is the predominant organism on skin commonly seen as a blood culture contaminant?

a. α-hemolytic streptococci
b. *B. fragilis*
c. *E. coli*
d. *Lactobacillus*
e. *S. epidermidis*

271. Which of the following is the predominant flora of the mouth that is the major cause of dental caries?

a. α-hemolytic streptococci
b. *B. fragilis*
c. *E. coli*
d. *Lactobacillus*
e. *S. epidermidis*

272. The bowel contains many microorganisms, but which of the following is the most prevalent bacterium?

a. α-hemolytic streptococci
b. *B. fragilis*
c. *E. coli*
d. *Lactobacillus*
e. *S. epidermidis*

273. Which of the following is the most prevalent microorganism in the vagina that may also be protective?

a. α-hemolytic streptococci
b. *B. fragilis*
c. *E. coli*
d. *Lactobacillus*
e. *S. epidermidis*

Questions 274–277

274. *Streptococcus mutans* is best described by which of the following statements?

a. An anaerobic, filamentous bacterium that often causes cervicofacial osteomyelitis
b. A β-hemolytic organism that causes a diffuse, rapidly spreading cellulitis
c. A facultative anaerobe that is highly cariogenic and sticks to teeth by synthesis of a dextran
d. A facultative anaerobe that often inhabits the buccal mucosa early in a neonate's life and can cause bacterial endocarditis
e. A facultatively anaerobic, rod-shaped bacterium that sticks to teeth and is cariogenic

275. *Streptococcus salivarius,* a common isolate in the clinical laboratory, is best described by which of the following statements?

a. An anaerobic, filamentous bacterium that often causes cervicofacial osteomyelitis
b. A β-hemolytic organism that causes a diffuse, rapidly spreading cellulitis
c. A facultative anaerobe that is highly cariogenic and sticks to teeth by synthesis of a dextran
d. A facultative anaerobe that often inhabits the buccal mucosa early in a neonate's life and can cause bacterial endocarditis
e. A facultatively anaerobic, rod-shaped bacterium that sticks to teeth and is cariogenic

276. *A. israelii* is one of many actinomycetes and is best described by which of the following statements?

a. An anaerobic, filamentous bacterium that often causes cervicofacial osteomyelitis
b. A β-hemolytic organism that causes a diffuse, rapidly spreading cellulitis
c. A facultative anaerobe that is highly cariogenic and sticks to teeth by synthesis of a dextran
d. A facultative anaerobe that often inhabits the buccal mucosa early in a neonate's life and can cause bacterial endocarditis
e. A facultatively anaerobic, rod-shaped bacterium that sticks to teeth and is cariogenic

277. *A. viscosus*, another ubiquitous actinomycete, can best be described by which of the following statements?

a. An anaerobic, filamentous bacterium that often causes cervicofacial osteomyelitis
b. A β-hemolytic organism that causes a diffuse, rapidly spreading cellulitis
c. A facultative anaerobe that is highly cariogenic and sticks to teeth by synthesis of a dextran
d. A facultative anaerobe that often inhabits the buccal mucosa early in a neonate's life and can cause bacterial endocarditis
e. A facultatively anaerobic, rod-shaped bacterium that sticks to teeth and is cariogenic

Questions 278–284

278. *C. diphtheriae* causes diphtheria, a rare disease in the United States. *C. diphtheriae* is best characterized by which of the following statements?

a. It produces at least one protein toxin consisting of two subunits, A and B, that cause severe spasmodic cough, usually in children
b. It produces a toxin that blocks protein synthesis in an infected cell and carries a lytic bacteriophage that produces the genetic information for toxin production
c. It secretes an erythrogenic toxin that causes the characteristic signs of scarlet fever
d. It secretes an exotoxin that has been called "verotoxin" and "Shiga-like toxin"; infection is mediated by specific attachment to mucosal membranes
e. It requires cysteine for growth

279. *Bordetella pertussis* is a gram-negative rod that causes severe respiratory disease. Which one of the following statements best characterizes this microorganism?

a. It produces at least one protein toxin consisting of two subunits, A and B, that cause severe spasmodic cough, usually in children
b. It produces a toxin that blocks protein synthesis in an infected cell and carries a lytic bacteriophage that produces the genetic information for toxin production
c. It secretes an erythrogenic toxin that causes the characteristic signs of scarlet fever
d. It secretes an exotoxin that has been called "verotoxin" and "Shiga-like toxin"; infection is mediated by specific attachment to mucosal membranes
e. It requires cysteine for growth

280. *F. tularensis* is the bacterium that causes tularemia, a disease not uncommonly seen in hunters. Which one of the following statements best characterizes this bacterium?

a. It produces at least one protein toxin consisting of two subunits, A and B, that cause severe spasmodic cough, usually in children
b. It produces a toxin that blocks protein synthesis in an infected cell and carries a lytic bacteriophage that produces the genetic information for toxin production
c. It secretes an erythrogenic toxin that causes the characteristic signs of scarlet fever
d. It secretes an exotoxin that has been called "verotoxin" and "Shiga-like toxin"; infection is mediated by specific attachment to mucosal membranes
e. It requires cysteine for growth

281. *E. coli* 0157/H7 is a newsworthy microorganism that has been isolated from foods (meat) and beverages (cider) with increasing frequency. Its characteristic biology is best described by which of the following statements?

a. It produces at least one protein toxin consisting of two subunits, A and B, that cause severe spasmodic cough, usually in children
b. It produces a toxin that blocks protein synthesis in an infected cell and carries a lytic bacteriophage that produces the genetic information for toxin production
c. It secretes an erythrogenic toxin that causes the characteristic signs of scarlet fever
d. It secretes an exotoxin that has been called "verotoxin" and "Shiga-like toxin"; infection is mediated by specific attachment to mucosal membranes
e. It requires cysteine for growth

282. *Streptococcus pyogenes* is a toxigenic bacterium causing a variety of diseases. Which of the following statements best characterizes this organism?

a. It produces at least one protein toxin consisting of two subunits, A and B, that cause severe spasmodic cough, usually in children
b. It produces a toxin that blocks protein synthesis in an infected cell and carries a lytic bacteriophage that produces the genetic information for toxin production
c. It secretes an erythrogenic toxin that causes the characteristic signs of scarlet fever
d. It secretes an exotoxin that has been called "verotoxin" and "Shiga-like toxin"; infection is mediated by specific attachment to mucosal membranes
e. It has capsules of polyglutamic acid, which is toxic when injected into rabbits

283. *N. meningitidis* causes meningitis in all age groups. Which of the following is a characteristic physiological trait?

a. It causes spontaneous abortion and has tropism for placental tissue due to the presence of erythritol in allantoic and amniotic fluid
b. It has a capsule of polyglutamic acid, which is toxic when injected into rabbits
c. It possesses N-acetylneuraminic acid capsule and adheres to specific tissues by pili found on the bacterial cell surface
d. It secretes two toxins, A and B, in the large bowel during antibiotic therapy
e. It synthesizes protein toxin as a result of colonization of vaginal tampons

284. *Brucella* is pathogenic for humans and animals. Which one of the following statements best characterizes this organism?

a. It causes spontaneous abortion and has tropism for placental tissue due to the presence of erythritol in allantoic and amniotic fluid
b. It has a capsule of polyglutamic acid, which is toxic when injected into rabbits
c. It has 82 polysaccharide capsular types; capsule is antiphagocytic; type 3 capsule (b-d-glucuronic acid polymer) most commonly seen in infected adults
d. It secretes two toxins, A and B, in the large bowel during antibiotic therapy
e. It synthesizes protein toxin as a result of colonization of vaginal tampons

Item 285–289

An 18-year-old male patient appeared at the emergency room with a three-day history of fever, dry cough, difficulty breathing, and muscle aches and pains. His chest x-ray showed a diffuse left upper lobe infiltrate. The following five questions focus on the etiology of "atypical" or community-acquired pneumonia.

285. *M. pneumoniae* pneumonia (walking pneumonia) may be rapidly identified by which of the following procedures?

a. Cold agglutinin test
b. Culture of respiratory secretions in HeLa cells after centrifugation of the inoculated tubes
c. Culture of respiratory secretions on monkey kidney cells
d. Detection of specific antigen in urine
e. Electron microscopy of sputum

286. Influenza can be treated; therefore, specific detection of the virus becomes much more important. Which of the following would be best for detection of influenza?

a. Cold agglutinin test
b. Culture of respiratory secretions on monkey kidney cells
c. Detection of antigen in respiratory secretions
d. Detection of specific antigen in urine
e. Electron microscopy of sputum

287. Legionnaires' disease is most rapidly diagnosed by which one of the following procedures?

a. Cold agglutinin test
b. Culture of respiratory secretions on a charcoal-based nutrient agar
c. Detection of antigen in respiratory secretions
d. Detection of specific antigen in urine
e. Electron microscopy of sputum

288. *Chlamydia pneumoniae* has recently been implicated in respiratory disease primarily in children. Which of the following would best isolate this fastidious bacterium?

a. Cold agglutinin test
b. Culture of respiratory secretions in HeLa cells after centrifugation of the inoculated tubes
c. Culture of respiratory secretions on monkey kidney cells
d. Detection of specific antigen in urine
e. Electron microscopy of sputum

289. *Bordetella* bronchitis, sometimes called whooping cough, can best be detected by which of the following procedures?

a. Cold agglutinin test
b. Culture of respiratory secretions in HeLa cells after centrifugation of the inoculated tubes
c. Culture of respiratory secretions on Regan-Lowe agar
d. Direct microscopy of sputum by Gram stain
e. Fluorescent antibody detection of the organism in sputum

Bacteriology

Answers

178. The answer is d. (*Brooks, pp 240–242. Levinson, p 128. Murray— 2002, pp 292–294. Ryan, pp 381–383.*) *H. pylori* was first recognized as a possible cause of gastritis and peptic ulcer by Marshall and Warren in 1984. This organism is readily isolated from gastric biopsies but not from stomach contents. It is similar to *Campylobacter* species and grows on chocolate agar at 37°C in the same microaerophilic environment suitable for *C. jejuni* (Campy-Pak or anaerobic jar [Gas Pak] without the catalyst). *H. pylori*, however, grows more slowly than *C. jejuni*, requiring five to seven days' incubation. *C. jejuni* grows optimally at 42°C, not 37°C, as does *H. pylori*.

Diagnostic Tests for *Helicobacter pylori*		
	Advantages	**Disadvantages**
Noninvasive		
Serum ELISA	Inexpensive	Not useful for follow-up
Urea breath test	Useful for follow-up	Expensive; may be falsely negative in patients on acid suppression therapy
Stool antigen test	Inexpensive; useful for follow-up	Inconvenient
Whole blood assay	Inexpensive; rapid	Less accurate than serum ELISA*
Invasive (endoscopic)		
Histology	Visualization of pathology	May miss low-grade infection
Rapid urease	Rapid	May be falsely positive in bacterial overgrowth
Culture	Antibiotic susceptibility	Not maximally sensitive; not available routinely; requires 4–7 d

*Enzyme-linked immunosorbent assay.

Reprinted, with permission, from Wilson WR, Sande MA. Current Diagnosis and Treatment in Infectious Disease. *New York: McGraw-Hill, 2001, 584.*

179. The answer is a. *(Brooks, pp 242–244. Levinson, pp 133–134. Murray—2002, pp 317–320. Ryan, pp 399–400.)* The major determinant of virulence in *H. influenzae* is the presence of a capsule. There is no demonstrable exotoxin, and the role of endotoxin is unclear. While one would expect that IgA protease would inhibit local immunity, the role of this enzyme in pathogenesis is as yet unclear.

180. The answer is e. *(Brooks, pp 221–222, 236. Levinson, pp 119, 126. Murray—2002, pp 269, 281–283. Ryan, pp 348, 375.)* The toxin of *V. cholerae* and LT enterotoxin from *E. coli* are similar. The B subunits of the toxins bind to ganglioside GM1 receptors on the host cell. The A subunits catalyze transfer of the ADP-ribose moiety of ADP to a regulatory protein known as G_s. This activated G_s stimulates adenyl cyclase. Cyclic AMP is increased, as is fluid and electrolyte release from the crypt cells into the lumen of the bowel. Watery, profuse diarrhea ensues.

181. The answer is d. *(Brooks, pp 272, 613. Levinson, p 158. Murray—2002, p 424. Ryan, p 904.)* Microscopic examination can readily demonstrate clue cells (epithelial cells with *Gardnerella* bacteria attached) as pseudohyphae (*Candida*). A wet mount will be needed to demonstrate motile *Trichomonas* cells. *Candida*, *Trichomonas*, and bacterial vaginitis are seen most often. *S. aureus* is involved much less frequently. While *E. coli* may be a common cause of genitourinary infection, clue cells are usually absent.

182. The answer is d. *(Brooks, pp 200–202. Levinson, pp 91–93. Murray—2002, p 213. Ryan, p 268.)* *S. aureus* is a well-known pathogen that is very opportunistic and commonly causes abscess lesions. It routinely may resist phagocytosis by white blood cells due to protein A. Osteomyelitis and arthritis, either hematogenous or traumatic, are commonly caused by *S. aureus,* especially in children. *Salmonella* are gram-negative. *S. saprophyticus* is a common skin flora and is usually not pathogenic. *S. pneumoniae* is seldom or never involved in osteomyelitis infections, as is true for *L. monocytogenes.*

183. The answer is c. *(Brooks, p 253. Levinson, p 141. Murray—2002, pp 322–323. Ryan, p 490.)* *Pasteurella* (gram-negative coccobacilli) are primarily animal pathogens, but they can cause a wide range of human diseases. They have a bipolar appearance on satined smears. *P. multocida* occurs worldwide in domestic and wild animals. It is the most common organism

GRAM-NEGATIVE RODS ASSOCIATED WITH THE RESPIRATORY TRACT

Species	Major Diseases	Laboratory Diagnosis	Factors X and V Required for Growth	Vaccine Available	Prophylaxis for Contacts
H. influenzae	Meningitis*; otitis media, sinusitis, pneumonia, epiglottitis	Culture; capsular polysaccharide in serum or spinal fluid	+	+	Rifampin
B. pertussis	Whooping cough (pertussis)	Fluorescent antibody on secretions; culture	–	+	Erythromycin
L. pneumophila	Pneumonia	Serology; urinary antigen; culture	–	–	None

*In countries where the H. influenzae b conjugate vaccine has been deployed, the vaccine has greatly reduced the incidence of meningitis caused by this organism.
Reprinted, with permission, from Levinson W, Jawetz E. Medical Microbiology and Immunology; 7e. New York: McGraw-Hill, 2002.

CLINICAL FEATURES OF VAGINITIS

	Normal	Vulvovaginal Candidiasis	Trichomoniasis	Bacterial Vaginosis
Symptoms	None	Pruritus Soreness Dyspareunia	Soreness Dyspareunia Often asymptomatic	Often asymptomatic Occasional abdominal pain
Discharge				
Amount	Variable	Scant/moderate	Profuse	Moderate
Color	Clear/white	White	Green-yellow	White/gray
Consistency	Nonhomogenous floccular	Clumped, adherent	Homogenous, frothy	Homogenous adherent
Vaginal fluid pH	4.0–4.5	4.0–4.5	5.0–6.0	>4.5
Amine test (fish odor)	None	None	Usually positive	Positive
Microscopy				
Saline	PMN:EC* ratio <1 Lactobacilli predominate	PMN:EC <1 Pseudohyphae (~40%)	PMN:EC >1 Motile trichomonads PMNs predominate	PMN:EC <1 Clue cells Coccobacilli
10% KOH	Negative	Pseudohyphae (~70%)	Negative	Negative

*PMN-Polymorphonuclear leukocytes; EC-vaginal epithelial cells.

Reprinted, with permission, from Wilson WR, Sande MA. Current Diagnosis and Treatment in Infectious Disease. New York: McGraw-Hill, 2001, 209.

in human wounds inflicted by bites of cats and dogs. It is a common cause of hemorrhagic septicemia in a variety of animals. Wounds commonly present with an acute onset, within hours, of redness, swelling, and pain. The other organisms are routinely found in the environment and may be opportunistic pathogens. *P. multocida* is a gram-negative rod that usually responds to penicillin treatment.

184–186. The answers are 184-c, 185-a, 186-a. *(Brooks, pp 297–298. Levinson, pp 150–151. Murray—2002, pp 395–399. Ryan, pp 410–411.)* M. *pneumoniae* causes a respiratory infection known as primary atypical pneumonia, or walking pneumonia. Although disease caused by *M. pneumoniae* can be contracted year-round, thousands of cases occur during the winter months in all age groups. The disease, if untreated, will persist for two weeks or longer. Rare but serious side effects include cardiomyopathies and CNS complications. Infection with *M. pneumoniae* may be treated with either erythromycin or tetracycline. The organism lacks a cell wall and so is resistant to the penicillin and the cephalosporin groups of antibiotics.

Until recently, diagnostic tests have been of limited value. Up to 50% of cases may not show cold agglutinins, an insensitive and nonspecific acute-phase reactant. However, if cold agglutinins are present, a quick diagnosis can be made if signs and symptoms are characteristic. Complement fixation tests that measure an antibody to a glycolipid antigen of *M. pneumoniae* are useful but not routinely performed in most laboratories. Also, cross-reactions may occur. Culture of *M. pneumoniae,* while not technically difficult, may take up to two weeks before visible growth is observed. A DNA probe is available. It is a 125I probe for the 16S ribosomal RNA of *M. pneumoniae*. Evaluations in a number of laboratories indicate that compared with culture it is highly sensitive and specific. Recently, DNA probes have been applied to the detection of *M. pneumoniae* in clinical specimens.

187. The answer is a. *(Brooks, pp 277–278. Levinson, pp 142–143. Murray—2002, pp 368–369. Ryan, pp 445–446.)* Most cases of tuberculosis are caused when patients inhale droplet nuclei containing infectious organisms. While the bacilli are deposited on the alveolar spaces, they do not clog up the alveoli but are engulfed by macrophages. Tissue injury is not a result of toxin secretion but of cell-mediated hypersensitivity, that is, "immunologic injury."

188. The answer is c. (*Brooks, p 171. Levinson, pp 67–68. Murray—2002, pp 192–193. Ryan, p 33.*) A new class of antibiotics, the quinolones, has one member, nalidixic acid, that has been available for years. The new representatives are much more active biologically and are effective against virtually all gram-negative bacteria and most gram-positive bacteria. They include norfloxacin, ofloxacin, ciprofloxacin, enoxacin, and the fluorinated quinolones such as lomefloxacin. These antibiotics kill bacteria by inhibition of synthesis of nucleic acid, more specifically, DNA gyrase. Resistance to quinolones has been observed and appears to be a class-specific phenomenon. An exception is when an organism is resistant to nalidixic acid, elevated minimal inhibitory concentrations (MICs) will generally apply to other quinolones, although these MICs will still be within the range of susceptibility.

189. The answer is c. (*Brooks, p 198. Levinson, p 76. Murray—2002, pp 215–216. Ryan, pp 269–270.*) Vancomycin-indeterminate *S. aureus* (VISA) was first recognized in Japan. Emergence in the United States soon followed. It is likely that the human VISA isolates have resulted from increased use of vancomycin for patients with MRSA or perhaps an increased pool of VISA in the environment selected out by the use of glycopeptides such as avoparcin, a growth promoter used in food-producing animals. In patients with VISA, the Centers for Disease Control (CDC) strongly recommends compliance with isolation procedures and other infection control practices geared to control of VISA.

190. The answer is a. (*Brooks, pp 611–612. Levinson, pp 28, 50–51. Murray—2002, p 322. Ryan, pp 854–855.*) Many sputum specimens are cultured unnecessarily. Sputum is often contaminated with saliva or is almost totally made up of saliva. These specimens rarely reveal the cause of the patient's respiratory problem and may provide laboratory information that is harmful. The sputum in the question appears to be a good specimen because there are few epithelial cells. The pleomorphic, gram-negative rods are suggestive of *Haemophilus*, but culture of the secretions is necessary. Normal flora from a healthy oral cavity consists of gram-positive cocci and rods, with few or no PMNs.

191. The answer is b. (*Brooks, p 267. Levinson, pp 131–132. Murray—2002, pp 356–357. Ryan, pp 324–325.*) *B. fragilis* is a constituent of normal intestinal flora and readily causes wound infections often mixed with aerobic isolates. These anaerobic, gram-negative rods are uniformly resistant to aminoglycosides and usually to penicillin as well. Reliable laboratory identification may require multiple analytical techniques. Generally, wound exudates smell bad owing to production of organic acids by such anaerobes as *B. fragilis.* Black exudates or a black pigment (heme) in the isolated colony is usually a characteristic of *Bacteroides* (*Porphyromonas*) *melaninogenicus,* not *B. fragilis.* Potent neurotoxins are synthesized by the gram-positive anaerobes such as *C. tetani* and *C. botulinum.*

192. The answer is b. (*Brooks, pp 255–257. Levinson, pp 105–106. Murray—2002, pp 257–258. Ryan, p 336.*) Typical *Neisseria* are gram-negative diplococci. *N. gonorrhoeae* contain pili, hairlike appendages that may be several micrometers long. They enhance attachment of the organism to mucous membranes, helping to make the organism more resistant to phagocytosis by white blood cells. Gonococci isolated from clinical specimens produce small colonies containing piliated bacteria. Capsules appear to be less important in gonococcal infection than *N. meningitidis* infections. Flagella, peptidoglycan, LPS, and F pili do not significantly relate to pathogenesis, other than that LPS (endotoxin) release may become significant later in infection.

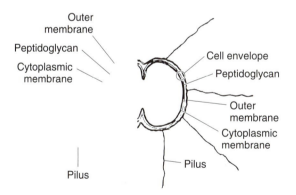

Collage and drawing of *N. gonorrhoeae* showing pili and the three layers of the cell envelope. (*Reproduced, with permission, from Brooks GF et al.* Jawetz's Medical Microbiology, *22e. New York: McGraw-Hill, 2001, 256.*)

193. The answer is b. *(Brooks, pp 192–193. Levinson, p 114. Murray—2002, pp 245–247. Ryan, pp 302–304.)* *Listeria* multiply both extracellularly and intracellularly, but under most circumstances a competent immune system eliminates *Listeria*. As expected, listeriosis is seen in the very young and the very old, and in people with compromised immune systems. Reports of *Listeria* food outbreaks have implicated such foods as coleslaw and milk products, especially if not pasteurized.

194–197. The answers are 194-d, 195-a, 196-c, 197-d. *(Brooks, pp 285–288. Levinson, pp 153–155. Murray—2002, pp 380–382. Ryan, pp 424–430.)* This patient appears to have primary syphilis, as evidenced by a penile chancre that was not tender. One of the differences between syphilis and herpes simplex virus (HSV) is that an HSV lesion is excruciatingly painful. Treponemal organisms may be seen microscopically in the lesion if the lesion is scraped. If not treated, the chancre will disappear and the patient will be asymptomatic until he/she exhibits the signs/symptoms of secondary syphilis, which include a disseminated rash and systemic involvement such as meningitis, hepatitis, or nephritis. There are two kinds of tests for the detection of syphilis antibodies: nonspecific tests such as the RPR and VDRL, and specific tests such as the FTA, TPHA (*T. pallidum* hemagglutination test), and the MHTP (microhemagglutination—*T. pallidum*). The difference is that the nonspecific tests use a cross-reactive antigen known as cardiolipin, while the specific tests use a *T. pallidum* antigen. Although the nonspecific tests are sensitive, they lack specificity and often cross-react in patients who have diabetes, hepatitis, or infectious mononucleosis, or who are pregnant. Some patients, especially those with autoimmune diseases, will have both nonspecific (RPR) and specific tests (FTA) positive even if they do not have syphilis. Resolution of such a situation can be done by molecular methods for *T. pallidum*, such as PCR, or by the immobilization test using live spirochetes and the patient's serum. In the TPI test, the spirochetes will die in the presence of specific antibody.

198. The answer is c. *(Brooks, pp 270–272. Levinson, pp 136, 137. Murray—2002, pp 325–327. Ryan, pp 415–419.)* The symptoms of Legionnaires' disease are similar to those of mycoplasmal pneumonia and influenza. Affected persons are moderately febrile, complain of pleuritic chest pain, and have a dry cough. Unlike *Klebsiella* and *Staphylococcus*, *L. pneumophila* exhibits fas-

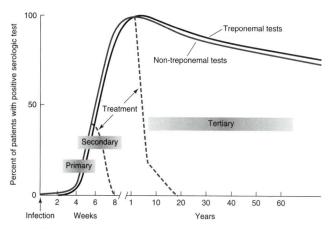

Treponemal and nontreponemal tests in syphilis. The time course of treated and un-treated syphilis in relation to serologic tests is shown. The nontreponemal tests (VDRL, RPR) rise during primary syphilis and reach their peak in secondary syphilis. They slowly decline with advancing age. With treatment they revert to normal over a few weeks. The treponemal tests (FTA-Abs, MHTP) follow the same course but remain elevated even following successful treatment. (*Reprinted, with permission, from Ryan KJ et al. Sherris Medical Microbiology, 4e. New York: McGraw-Hill, 2001, 429.*)

tidious growth requirements. Charcoal yeast extract agar either with or without antibiotics is the preferred isolation medium. While sputum may not be the specimen of choice for *Legionella,* the discovery of small, gram-negative rods by direct fluorescent antibody (FA) technique should certainly heighten suspicion of the disease. *L. pneumophila* is a facultative intracellular pathogen and enters macrophages without activating their oxidizing capabilities. The organisms bind to macrophage C receptors, which promote engulfment.

199. The answer is b. (*Brooks, p 187. Levinson, pp 111–112. Murray— 2002, pp 349–351. Ryan, pp 322–324.*) Patients treated with antibiotics develop diarrhea that, in most cases, is self-limiting. However, in some instances, particularly in those patients treated with ampicillin or clindamycin, a severe, life-threatening pseudomembranous enterocolitis develops. This disease has characteristic histopathology, and membranous plaques can be seen in the colon by endoscopy. Pseudomembranous enterocolitis and antibiotic-associated diarrhea are caused by an anaerobic gram-positive rod, *C. difficile.* It has been recently shown that *C. difficile* produces a protein toxin with a molecular weight of about 250,000. The "toxin" is, in fact, two toxins, toxin A and toxin B. Both toxins are always present in fecal samples, but there is approximately 1000 times more toxin B than toxin A. Toxin A has enterotoxic activity—that is, it elicits a positive fluid response in ligated rabbit ileal loops—whereas toxin B appears to be primarily a cytotoxin.

200. The answer is b. *(Brooks, pp 192–193, 207. Levinson, pp 95, 114. Murray—2002, p 226, 246. Ryan, pp 286–287, 302–305.)* Group B streptococci are normal flora in a sizeable number of women, who show no vaginal adverse disease. *L. monocytogenes* also may be present as normal vaginal flora. Streptococci from clinical specimens usually grow in small, pinpoint colonies. *Listeria,* usually growing intracellularly in vivo, also produce small colonies on blood agar. Both also produce β (clear zone) hemolysis. Of the proposed tests, catalase is easy to perform and interpret. Group B streptococci do not produce catalase, while *Listeria* are catalase-positive.

STREPTOCOCCI OF MEDICAL IMPORTANCE			
Species	**Lancefield Group**	**Typical Hemolysis**	**Diagnostic Features[1]**
S. pyogenes	A	β	Bacitracin-sensitive
S. agalactiae	B	β	Bacitracin-resistant; hippurate hydrolyzed
E. faecalis	D	α or β or none	Growth in 6.5% NaCl[3]
S. bovis[2]	D	α or none	No growth in 6.5% NaCl
S. pneumoniae	NA[4]	α	Bile-soluble; inhibited by optochin
Viridans group[5]	NA	α	Not bile-soluble; not inhibited by optochin

[1]All streptococci are catalase-negative.
[2]*S. bovis* is a nonenterococcal group D organism.
[3]Both *E. faecalis* and *S. bovis* grow on bile-esculin agar, whereas other streptococci do not. They hydrolyze the esculin, and this results in a characteristic black discoloration of the agar.
[4]NA, not applicable.
[5]Viridans group streptococci include several species, such as *S. anguis, S. mutans, S. mitis, S. gordoni, S. salivarius, S. anginosus, S. milleri,* and *S. intermedius.*

Reprinted, with permission, from Levinson W, Jawetz E. Medical Microbiology and Immunology, 7e. New York: McGraw-Hill, 2002, 95.

201. The answer is a. *(Brooks, pp 242–244. Levinson, pp 133–134. Murray—2002, p 319. Ryan, pp 397–401.)* Meningitis caused by H. *influenzae* cannot be distinguished on clinical grounds from that caused by pneumococci or meningococci. The symptoms described are typical for all three organisms. H. *influenzae* is a small, gram-negative rod with a polysaccharide capsule. It is able to grow on laboratory media if two factors are added. Heme (factor X) and NAD (factor V) provide for energy production. Use of the conjugate vaccine (type b polysaccharide) reduces the disease incidence more than 90%. Pneumococci are gram-positive diplococci, and meningococci are gram-negative diplococci, which grow on blood agar and chocolate agar with no X and V factors needed, respectively.

202. The answer is a. *(Brooks, pp 194–196. Levinson, pp 149–150. Murray—2002, pp 335–337. Ryan, pp 458–459.)* The patient presented with typical symptoms of actinomycosis. A. *israelii* is normal flora in the mouth. However, it causes a chronic draining infection, often around the maxilla or the mandible, with osteomyelitic changes. Treatment is high-dose penicillin for four to six weeks. The diagnosis of actinomycosis is often complicated by the failure of A. *israelii* to grow from the clinical specimen. It is an obligate anaerobe. Fluorescent antibody (FA) reagents are available for direct staining of A. *israelii*. A rapid diagnosis can be made from the pus. FA conjugates are also available for A. *viscosus* and *Actinomyces odontolyticus*, anaerobic actinomycetes that are rarely involved in actinomycotic abscesses.

203–205. The answers are 203-a, 204-b, 205-b. *(Brooks, pp 192–193. Levinson, p 95. Murray—2002, p 226. Ryan, pp 286–287.)* The incidence of group B streptococcal (GBS) disease is 1 to 3 cases per 1000 births. Neonates acquire the disease during birth from mothers who harbor the organism. Risk factors include prematurity, premature rupture of membranes, and group B streptococcal carriage. The Gram stain of cerebrospinal fluid is a rapid test for GBS disease. Although sensitive, the Gram stain requires experience to differentiate these streptococci from other gram-positive cocci. Latex tests for GBS antigen are also available, but sensitivity in CSF is not significantly higher than the Gram stain. GBS can be reduced by intrapartum administration of penicillin. While GBS is relatively more resistant to penicillin than group A streptococci, the great majority of GBS isolates are still penicillin-susceptible. An aminoglycoside such as gentamicin may be added to GBS treatment regimens due to the relative reduced susceptibility of some strains. Experimentally, GBS polysaccharide vaccines have also been used. Screening pregnant females early in pregnancy probably offers little advantage because of the possible acquisition of GBS late in the pregnancy. There has been speculation concerning the pathogenesis of GBS. This includes failure to activate complement pathways and immobilization of polymorphonuclear leukocytes due to the inactivation of complement C5a, a potent chemoattractant.

206. The answer is a. (*Brooks, pp 285–288. Levinson, pp 153–155. Murray— 2002, pp 381–383. Ryan, pp 424–429.*) In men, the appearance of a hard chancre on the penis characteristically indicates syphilis. Even though the chancre does not appear until the infection is two or more weeks old, the VDRL test for syphilis still can be negative despite the presence of a chancre (the VDRL test may not become positive for two or three weeks after initial infection). However, a lesion suspected of being a primary syphilitic ulcer should be examined by dark-field microscopy, which can reveal motile treponemes.

207. The answer is a. (*Brooks, pp 246–248. Levinson, pp 138–139. Murray— 2002, pp 312–313. Ryan, pp 483–484.*) *Brucella* are small, aerobic, gram-negative coccobacilli. Of the four well-characterized species of *Brucella*, only one—*B. melitensis*—characteristically infects both goats and humans. Brucellosis may be associated with gastrointestinal and neurologic symptoms, lymphadenopathy, splenomegaly, hepatitis, and osteomyelitis. Susceptibility to dyes (thionin and basic fuschin) can help in differentiation of the species.

GRAM-NEGATIVE RODS ASSOCIATED WITH ANIMAL SOURCES				
Species	**Disease**	**Source of Human Infection**	**Mode of Transmission from Animal to Human**	**Diagnosis**
Brucella species	Brucellosis	Pigs, cattle, goats, sheep	Dairy products; contact with animal tissues	Serology or culture
F. tularensis	Tularemia	Rabbits, deer, ticks	Contact with animal tissues; ticks	Serology
Y. pestis	Plague	Rodents	Flea bite	Immunofluorescence or culture
P. multocida	Cellulitis	Cats, dogs	Cat or dog bite	Wound culture

Reprinted, with permission, from Levinson W, Jawetz E. Medical Microbiology and Immunology, 7e. New York: McGraw-Hill, 2002, 139.

SPIROCHETES OF MEDICAL IMPORTANCE

Species	Disease	Mode of Transmission	Diagnosis	Morphology	Growth in Bacteriologic Media	Treatment
T. pallidum	Syphilis	Intimate (sexual) contact; across the placenta	Microscopy; serologic tests	Thin, tight, spirals, seen by dark-field illumination, silver impregnation, or immunofluorescent stain	—	Penicillin G
B. burgdorferi	Lyme disease	Tick bite	Clinical observations; microscopy	Large, loosely coiled; stain with Giemsa stain	+	Tetracycline or amoxicillin for acute; penicillin G for chronic
B. recurrentis	Relapsing fever	Louse bite	Clinical observations; microscopy	Large, loosely coiled; stain with Giemsa stain	+	Tetracycline
L. interrogans	Leptospirosis	Food or drink contaminated by urine of infected animals (rats, dogs, pigs, cows)	Serologic tests	Thin, tight spirals, seen by dark-field illumination	+	Penicillin G

Reprinted, with permission, from Levinson W, Jawetz E. Medical Microbiology and Immunology, 7e. New York: McGraw-Hill, 2002, 154.

208. The answer is a. *(Brooks, pp 235–237. Levinson, pp 125–126. Murray—2002, pp 284–286. Ryan, pp 376–377.)* Cholera is a toxicosis. The mode of action of cholera toxin is to stimulate the activity of adenyl cyclase, an enzyme that converts ATP to cyclic AMP. Cyclic AMP stimulates the secretion of chloride ion, and affected patients lose copious amounts of fluid. A drug that inhibits adenyl cyclase thus might block the effect of cholera toxin. Water and electrolyte replacement are primary management mechanisms, while oral tetracycline may help reduce stool output.

209. The answer is d. *(Brooks, pp 200–201. Levinson, pp 93–94. Murray—2002, pp 209–211. Ryan, pp 263–264.)* Certain strains of staphylococci elaborate an enterotoxin that is frequently responsible for food poisoning. Typically, the toxin is produced when staphylococci grow on foods rich in carbohydrates and is present in the food when it is consumed. The resulting gastroenteritis is dependent only on the ingestion of toxin and not on bacterial multiplication in the gastrointestinal tract. Characteristic symptoms are nausea, vomiting, abdominal cramps, and explosive diarrhea. The illness rarely lasts more than 24 hours.

210. The answer is e. *(Brooks, p 198. Levinson, p 91. Murray—2002, p 207. Ryan, pp 269–270.)* Staphylococci are gram-positive, non-spore-forming cocci. Clinically, their antibiotic resistance poses major problems. Many strains produce β-lactamase (penicillinase), an enzyme that destroys penicillin by opening the lactam ring. Drug resistance, mediated by plasmids, may be transferred by transduction.

211. The answer is c. *(Brooks, pp 183–184. Levinson, p 110. Murray—2002, pp 347–349. Ryan, pp 320–322.)* C. botulinum growing in food produces a potent neurotoxin that causes diplopia, dysphagia, respiratory paralysis, and speech difficulties when ingested by humans. The toxin is thought to act by blocking the action of acetylcholine at neuromuscular junctions. Botulism is associated with high mortality; fortunately, *C. botulinum* infection in humans is rare.

212. The answer is a. *(Brooks, pp 262–263. Levinson, pp 103–106. Murray—2002, p 265. Ryan, p 327.)* Several *Neisseria* species make up part of the normal (nonpathogenic) flora of the human upper respiratory tract. While commensal organisms seldom cause disease, they may occasionally be opportunistic. These organisms are also "foreign" to the immune system and cause immune responses to occur, especially humoral (antibody). The pathogens (*N. gonorrhae* and *N. meningitidis*) produce factors that ensure successful colonization of tissue in spite of local immune defense mechanisms.

213. The answer is d. (*Brooks, pp 239–244. Levinson, pp 127–128. Murray—2002, pp 288–289. Ryan, pp 379–380.*) Until recently, both erythromycin and ciprofloxacin were the drugs of choice for *C. jejuni* enterocolitis. Recently, resistance to the quinolones (ciprofloxacin) has been observed. Ampicillin is ineffective against this gram-negative, curved rod. While Pepto-Bismol may be adequate for a related ulcer-causing bacterium, *Helicobacter*, it is not used for *C. jejuni*. While the pathogenesis of *C. jejuni* suggests an enterotoxin, an antitoxin is not available.

214. The answer is b. (*Brooks, pp 242–244. Levinson, pp 133–134. Murray—2002, pp 317–318. Ryan, pp 397–401.*) *H. influenzae* is a gram-negative bacillus. In young children, it can cause pneumonitis, sinusitis, otitis, and meningitis. Occasionally, it produces a fulminative laryngotracheitis with such severe swelling of the epiglottis that tracheostomy becomes necessary. Clinical infections with this organism after the age of three years are less frequent, especially since approval of the type b vaccine.

215–217. The answers are 215-a, 216-d, 217-e. (*Brooks, pp 214–215. Levinson, pp 98, 100. Murray—2002, pp 236–238. Ryan, pp 294–295.*) Enterococci cause a wide variety of infections ranging from less serious—for example, urinary tract infections—to very serious, such as septicemia. A gram-positive coccus resistant to penicillin must be assumed to be enterococcus until other, more definitive biochemical testing places the isolate in one of the more esoteric groups of gram-positive cocci. Once isolated, there are a variety of tests to speciate enterococci. However, penicillin-resistant, non-β-lactamase-producing, vancomycin-resistant, gram-positive cocci are most likely *E. faecium*. There are a variety of mechanisms for vancomycin resistance in *E. faecium* and they have been termed Van A, B, or C. These isolates have become one of the most feared nosocomial pathogens in the hospital environment. Unfortunately, no approved antibiotics can successfully treat vancomycin-resistant enterococci (VRE)—only some experimental antibiotics such as Synercid.

218. The answer is c. (*Brooks, p 200. Levinson, p 91. Murray—2002, p 213. Ryan, p 824.*) *S. aureus* is implicated in the majority of cases of acute osteomyelitis, which affects children most often. A superficial staphylococcal lesion frequently precedes the development of bone infection. In the preantibiotic era, *S. pneumoniae* was a common cause of acute osteomyelitis. *M. tuberculosis* and gram-negative organisms are implicated less frequently in this infection.

219. The answer is c. (*Brooks, pp 188–191. Levinson, pp 112–113. Murray—2002, p 251. Ryan, p 170.*) All toxigenic strains of *C. diphtheriae* are lysogenic for β-phage carrying the Tox gene, which codes for the toxin molecule. The expression of this gene is controlled by the metabolism of the host bacteria. The greatest amount of toxin is produced by bacteria grown on media containing very low amounts of iron. Fragment B of the toxin is required for cell entry, while Fragment A stops protein production by inhibiting elongation factor 2.

220–222. The answers are 220-e, 221-d, 222-b. (*Brooks, p 201. Levinson, p 92. Murray—2002, p 211. Ryan, pp 264–266.*) Toxic shock syndrome (TSS) is a febrile illness seen predominantly, but not exclusively, in menstruating women. Clinical criteria for TSS include fever greater than 102°F (38.9°C), rash, hypotension, and abnormalities of the mucous membranes and the gastrointestinal, hepatic, muscular, cardiovascular, or central nervous system. Usually three or more systems are involved. Treatment is supportive, including the aggressive use of antistaphylococcal antibiotics. Certain types of tampons may play a role in TSS by trapping O_2 and depleting magnesium. Most people have protective antibodies to the toxic shock syndrome toxin (TSST-1).

TSS is caused by a toxin-producing strain of *S. aureus* (TSST-1). While there have been reports that *S. epidermidis* produces TSS, they have largely been discounted. Vaginal colonization with *S. aureus* is a necessary adjunct to the disease. *S. aureus* is isolated from the vaginal secretions, conjunctiva, nose, throat, cervix, and feces in 45 to 98% of cases. The organism has infrequently been isolated from the blood.

Epidemiologic investigations suggest strongly that toxic shock syndrome is related to use of tampons, in particular, use of the highly absorbent ones that can be left in for extended periods of time. An increased growth of intravaginal *S. aureus* and enhanced production of TSST-1 have been associated with the prolonged intravaginal use of these hyperabsorbent tampons and with the capacity of the materials used in them to bind magnesium. The most severe cases of TSS have been seen in association with gram-negative infection. TSST-1 may enhance endotoxin activity. Recently, group A streptococci have been reported to cause TSS.

223–224. The answers are 223-c, 224-d. Bayesian statistics are often used to determine sensitivity, specificity, and predictive values of new diagnostic tests. A square is set up and the experimental numbers inserted: a = true positive, b = false positive, c = false negative, and d = true negative. The formulas for sensitivity, specificity, and predictive values are also given.

It is necessary to note that the incidence of the disease in the population affects predictive values but not sensitivity or specificity. At a given level of sensitivity and specificity, as the incidence of the disease in the population increases, the predictive value of a positive (PVP) increases, and the predictive value of a negative (PVN) decreases. For this reason, predictive values are difficult to interpret unless true disease incidence is known.

	Culture	
LA Test	**Pos**	**Neg**
POS	(a) 25	(b) 5
NEG	(c) 5	(d) 95

$$\text{Sensitivity} = \frac{a}{a+c} = \frac{25}{25+5} = 85\%$$

$$\text{Specificity} = \frac{d}{d+b} = \frac{95}{95+5} = 95\%$$

$$\text{PVP} = \frac{a}{a+b} = \frac{25}{25+5} = 85\%$$

$$\text{PVN} = \frac{d}{d+c} = \frac{95}{95+5} = 95\%$$

225. The answer is d. (*Brooks, pp 229–230. Levinson, pp 130–131. Murray—2002, pp 297–300. Ryan, pp 387–388.*) Pseudomonads occur widely in soil, water, plants, and animals. They are gram-negative, motile, aerobic rods that produce water-soluble pigments (blue and green). They are very opportunistic when abnormal host defenses are encountered. While motile, they do not "swarm" over the surface of an agar plate, as *Proteus* does. Being gram-negative, as many enteric and environmental organisms are, their cell walls contain endotoxin (LPS). Many of the pseudomonads are resistant to a wide range of antimicrobials, enhancing their opportunistic characteristics.

226. The answer is c. (*Brooks, pp 182–183, 186–187. Levinson, pp 108, 110–111. Murray—2002, pp 243–244, 343–344. Ryan, pp 308, 314–317.*) *Clostridium* and *Bacillus* organisms exist widely in nature. While many *Clostridium* are pathogenic due to exotoxin production (*C. tetani, C. botulism*) and anthrax has multiple virulence factors (capsule, LF, EF, and PA), *C. perfringens* and *B. cereus* are found routinely in gastroenteritis outbreaks. Since both are sporeformers, the usual epidemiological investigation finds that heating foods kills vegetative bacteria but not spores. If food is inappropriately stored (>40°F–140°F), spores may germinate into vegetative bacteria and be ingested, causing the disease. Most episodes are self-limited. Both produce enterotoxins that account for similar disease presentations.

227. The answer is e. (*Brooks, p 198. Levinson, pp 94–95. Murray—2002, p 215. Ryan, pp 269–270.*) The incidence of oxacillin- and methicillin-resistant *S. aureus* (MRSA) has been rapidly increasing. MRSA and methicillin-sensitive *S. aureus* (MSSA) coexist in heterologous populations. Treatment of a patient harboring this heterologous population may provide a selective environment for the MRSA. Prior to changing therapy, the susceptibility of the isolate should be determined. Vancomycin has often been used effectively for MRSA, but it is expensive and nephrotoxic. There is no evidence that MRSA is any more virulent or invasive than susceptible strains.

STAPHYLOCOCCI OF MEDICAL IMPORTANCE				
Species	**Coagulase Production**	**Typical Hemolysis**	**Important Features***	**Typical Disease**
S. aureus	+	Beta	Protein A on surface	Abscess, food poisoning, toxic shock syndrome
S. epidermidis	−	None	Sensitive to novobiocin	Infection of prosthetic heart valves and hips; common member of skin flora
S. saprophyticus	−	None	Resistant to novobiocin	Urinary tract infection

*All staphylococci are catalase-positive.

Reprinted, with permission, from Levinson W, Jawetz E. Medical Microbiology and Immunology, 7e. New York: McGraw-Hill, 2002, 92.

228. The answer is b. (Levinson, pp 330–331. Murray—2002, pp 707–709.) Coccidian-like bodies have been identified in stools of some patients with diarrhea. These organisms appear to be similar to blue-green algae and were referred to as Cyanobacterium-like until they were recently reclassified as Cyclospora. They are larger than the microsporidia and resemble neither Giardia nor Prototheca nor other algae-like organisms. Unlike Cryptosporidium, these organisms fluoresce under ultraviolet light. The diarrhea can be prolonged and relapsing, and the treatment is usually trimethoprim-sulfamethoxazole.

229. The answer is c. (Brooks, pp 221–222. Levinson, pp 120–121. Murray—2002, pp 271–272. Ryan, pp 355–357.) Food poisoning with E. coli 0157/H7 causes hemorrhagic colitis; it is often seen in people who have eaten beef hamburgers. The same organism also causes a hemorrhagic uremic syndrome. The toxin, called Shiga-like toxin, can be demonstrated in Vero cells, but the cytotoxicity must be neutralized with specific antiserum. With the exception of sorbitol fermentation, there is nothing biochemically distinctive about these organisms.

230. The answer is b. (Brooks, pp 221–222. Levinson, pp 120–121. Murray—2002, pp 271–272. Ryan, pp 355–357.) LT and ST proteins are characteristic of enterotoxigenic E. coli. To cause diarrhea, E. coli must produce not only LT and ST toxins but also adhere to the lining of the small intestine. Fimbrial antigens are involved in adherence. O657/H7 stain is called enterohemorrhagic E. coli (EHEC), while enteropathogenic E. coli (EPEC) is also an important cause of diarrhea in infants. Enterotoxigenic E. coli (ETEC) is an important cause of traveler's diarrhea, producing a heat-labile exotoxin and a heat-stable enterotoxin. Enteroinvasive E. coli (EIEC) produces a shigellosis-type disease.

231. The answer is d. (Brooks, pp 250–251. Levinson, pp 140–141. Murray—2002, pp 276–278. Ryan, pp 484–488.) Bubonic plague and pneumonic plague differ clinically. Bubonic plague, characterized by swollen lymph nodes and fever, is usually transmitted through a flea bite. Pneumonic plague, which is characterized by sepsis and pneumonia, is transmitted by the droplet route, usually after contact with an infected human or animal.

232. The answer is a. (Brooks, p 273. Levinson, pp 165–166. Murray—2002, pp 329–330. Ryan, p 479.) While the essential information (i.e., the evidence that the child in question was scratched by a cat) is missing, the clinical presentation points to a number of diseases, including cat-scratch disease (CSD). Until recently, the etiologic agent of CSD was unknown. Evidence indicated that it was a pleomorphic, rod-shaped bacterium that had been named *Afipia*. It was best demonstrated in the affected lymph node by a silver impregnation stain. However, it now appears that *Afipia* causes relatively few cases of CSD and that the free-living rickettsia primarily responsible is *Rochalimaea henselae*, which has recently been renamed *Bartonella henselae*.

233. The answer is c. (*Brooks, p 208. Levinson, p 98. Murray—2002, p 222. Ryan, p 273.*) There has been a marked increase in fatal streptococcal infections, including those that are described as "necrotizing fasciitis." The strains of group A streptococci isolated have a pyrogenic exotoxin with properties not unlike those of the toxic shock toxin of *S. aureus*. Mortality is high (30%) in spite of aggressive antibiotic therapy.

234. The answer is b. (*Brooks, pp 240–241. Levinson, p 128. Murray—2002, pp 292–294. Ryan, pp 383–384.*) H. pylori antigen tests using an ELISA format and a monoclonal antibody to *H. pylori* are as sensitive as culture of the control portion of the stomach. Urea breath tests are also widely used. *H. pylori* has an active enzyme (urease) that breaks down radioactive urea. The patient releases radioactive CO_2 if *H. pylori* are present. *H. pylori* antibody tests, IgG and IgA, indicate the presence of *H. pylori* and usually decline after effective treatment. Culture of stomach contents is insensitive and not appropriate as a diagnostic procedure for *H. pylori*. Direct tests such as antigen or culture of gastric mucosa are preferred because they are the most sensitive indication of a cure.

235. The answer is c. (*Brooks, pp 290–291. Levinson, pp 155–157. Murray—2002, pp 389–390. Ryan, pp 434–437.*) At the present time, Lyme disease may be diagnosed clinically and serologically. Patients who are from endemic areas such as eastern Pennsylvania and report joint pain and swelling months subsequent to exposure to ticks must be evaluated for Lyme disease and treated if the test is positive. Patients may also report a variety of neurologic problems such as tingling of the extremities, Bell's palsy, and headache. IgM antibody appears soon after the tick bite (10 days to three weeks) and persists for two months; IgG appears later in the disease but remains elevated for one to two years, especially in untreated patients. A significant IgG titer is at least 1:320. Most investigators feel that IgM titers of 1:100 are significant; some investigators say that any IgM titer is significant.

236. The answer is c. *(Brooks, p 282. Levinson, p 147. Murray—2002, p 585. Ryan, p 613.)* There are some interesting characteristics of M. avium from AIDS patients. According to data from the National Jewish Hospital and Research Center in Denver and the Centers for Disease Control, 75% of the isolates were serovar 4, and 76% produced a deep-yellow pigment. Yellow pigment is not a characteristic of most isolates of M. avium. The significance of these findings is unknown. Most M. avium isolates are resistant to isoniazid and streptomycin but susceptible to clofazimine and ansamycin. In vitro susceptibility testing, however, may not be reliable for M. avium. A blood culture is often the most reliable way to diagnose the disease.

237. The answer is b. *(Brooks, pp 209–210. Levinson, p 99. Murray—2002, p 223. Ryan, p 279.)* Rheumatic fever (RF) is a disease that causes polyarthritis, carditis, chorea, and erythema marginatum. The mechanism of damage appears to be autoimmune; that is, antibodies are synthesized to a closely related streptococcal antigen such as M-protein, but these same antibodies cross-react with certain cardiac antigens such as myosin. Until recently, RF was very rare in the United States. In 1986, there were at least 135 cases of RF in Utah. Subsequently, scattered cases of RF have occurred in other states. Epidemiologists do not have a reason for this increase in RF. Some evidence suggests that there may be a genetic predisposition to the disease. Intramuscular injection of benzathine penicillin is effective treatment for and prophylaxis against group A streptococcal infection.

238. The answer is d. *(Brooks, p 209. Levinson, p 98. Murray—2002, pp 229–230. Ryan, pp 293–294.)* In the healthy oral cavity, gram-positive, α-hemolytic streptococci make up the predominant flora. Any dental manipulation causes bleeding, allowing the oral flora to get into the blood (bacteremia). Phagocytic activity by white blood cells usually clears this in a few minutes. However, these same organisms are quite efficient at attaching to and colonizing heart valve defects. S. viridians is a typical member of this α-hemolytic group and is commonly found in subacute bacterial endocarditis.

239. The answer is c. *(Brooks, pp 593–594. Levinson, pp 335–336. Murray—2002, pp 759–760. Ryan, pp 799–801.)* *Echinococcus* is a small, three-segmented tapeworm found only in the intestines of dogs and other carnivores. Eggs leave these hosts and infect grazing animals. In the herbivore gut, the eggs hatch and the released forms penetrate the gut. Various organs (especially the liver) develop huge, fluid-filled cysts in which future scoleces form (hydatid sand). Dogs become infected when they feed on viscera of diseased sheep or cows. Hydatid disease in humans occurs only through ingestion of dog feces. Humans are only an intermediate host of this organism and never the final host. None of the other options are cestodes, or tapeworms.

240. The answer is e. *(Brooks, pp 211–213. Levinson, pp 94–95. Murray—2002, pp 203–235. Ryan, p 291.)* The quellung test determines the presence of bacterial capsules. Specific antibody is mixed with the bacterial suspension or with clinical material. The polysaccharide capsule-antibody complex is visible microscopically. The test is also termed *capsular swelling*. The capsules of *S. pneumoniae* as well as *N. meningitidis*, *H. influenzae*, and *K. pneumoniae* play a role in the phatogenicity of the organisms. These surface structures inhibit phagocytosis, perhaps by preventing attachment of the leukocyte pseudopod. *C. diphtheriae*, *Enterobacter*, and *H. parainfluenzae* are nonencapsulated.

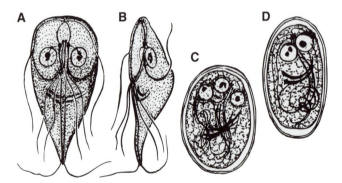

Giardia lamblia. A: "Face" and B: "profile" of vegetative forms; C and D: cysts (binucleate [D] and quadrinucleate stages). 2000 ×. *(Reproduced, with permission, from Brooks GF et al. Jawetz's Medical Microbiology, 22e. New York: McGraw-Hill, 2001, 562.)*

241. The answer is b. *(Brooks, pp 192–193. Levinson, p 114. Murray—2002, pp 245–247. Ryan, pp 302–305.)* Except during a meningococcal epidemic, *H. influenzae* is the most common cause of bacterial meningitis in children. The organism is occasionally found to be associated with respiratory tract infections or otitis media. *H. influenzae, N. meningitidis, S. pneumoniae,* and *Listeria* account for 80 to 90% of all cases of bacterial meningitis. A purified polysaccharide vaccine conjugated to protein for *H. influenzae* type B is available. A tetravalent vaccine is available for *N. meningitidis* and a 23-serotype vaccine for *S. pneumoniae.* No vaccine is available for *Listeria.*

242–245. The answers are 242-e, 243-d, 244-a, 245-b. *(Brooks, pp 137–140. Levinson, pp 29–33. Murray—2002, p 177.)* Organisms may be transmitted in a number of ways, such as by air, food, hands, sexual contact, and infected needles. However, for each disease or disease category, there is usually a portal of entry not always unique to the organism. The respiratory tract is a common portal of entry to such airborne organisms as *M. tuberculosis.* This is why respiratory precautions must be taken when patients are harboring viable *M. tuberculosis.* The gastrointestinal tract is usually infected from ingestion of contaminated food or water (*Shigella, Salmonella, Campylobacter*) or by an alteration of the normal microbial flora such as with *C. difficile* disease. The skin is a tough integument and, intact, is resistant to most infectious organisms except those that may break down human skin. Breaches of the skin as by wounds, burns, and the like predispose patients to a variety of infections such as tetanus caused by wound contamination with spores of *C. tetani,* or direct infection by *Staphylococcus, Streptococcus,* or gram-negative rods (such as *Serratia* or *Pseudomonas*). The genital tract may become infected either by sexual contact or by alteration of the genital environment, as often occurs with yeast infections. Several bacteria such as *N. gonorrhoeae, Chlamydia,* and *T. pallidum* are transmitted by direct sexual contact with infected partners.

246–247. The answers are 246-d, 247-b. *(Brooks, p 233, 262. Levinson, p 166, 168. Murray—2002, pp 303, 331. Ryan, pp 390–391.)* While admittedly rare in human medicine, the bacteria referred to should be appreciated for their role in human disease. *Branhamella* is a gram-negative diplococcus. It has recently been renamed *Moraxella catarrhalis.* While it is a member of the normal flora, it may cause severe upper and lower respiratory tract infection, particularly in the immunosuppressed patient. Most isolates produce β-lactamase and are resistant to penicillin. *Capnocytophaga* grows best in a carbon dioxide atmosphere, as the name implies. It is isolated frequently from patients with periodontal disease but may also cause septicemia in susceptible patients. Rat-bite fever is caused by *Spirillum,* and the agent of cat-scratch disease is *B. henselae.*

248. The answer is b. (*Brooks, pp 301–303. Levinson, pp 162–164. Murray—2002, pp 402–404. Ryan, pp 477–478.*) *Coxiella burnetii* is a rickettsial organism that causes upper respiratory infections in humans. These can range from subclinical infection to influenza-like disease and pneumonia. Transmission to humans occurs from inhalation of dust contaminated with rickettsiae from placenta, dried feces, urine, or milk, or from aerosols in slaughterhouses. *C. burnetii* can also be found in ticks, which can transmit the agent to sheep, goats, and cattle. No skin rash occurs in these infections. Treatment includes tetracycline and chloramphenicol.

249–251. The answers are 249-a, 250-d, 251-b. (*Brooks, pp 194–196, 214, 610. Levinson, pp 56, 100, 149. Murray—2002, pp 199–200, 236–238, 337. Ryan, pp 294, 457–459, 870–871.*) These questions demonstrate commonly occurring clinical infectious diseases and microbiologic problems. Enterococci may be resistant to ampicillin and gentamicin. Vancomycin would be the drug of choice. However, laboratory results do not always correlate well with clinical response. The National Committee on Clinical Laboratory Standards recommends testing enterococci only for ampicillin and vancomycin. Some symptomatic patients may have 10 leukocytes per mL of urine but relatively few bacteria. The patient is likely infected and the organisms, particularly if in pure culture, should be further processed.

The patient in question 251 probably has actinomycosis. These laboratory data are not uncommon. There is no reason to work up all the contaminating bacteria. A fluorescent microscopy test for *A. israelii* is available. If positive, the FA provides a rapid diagnosis. In any event, it may be impossible to recover *A. israelii* from such a specimen. High-dose penicillin has been used to treat actinomycosis.

252–256. The answers are 252-c, 253-d, 254-b, 255-d, 256-e. (*Brooks, pp 144–150. Levinson, pp 59–70. Murray—2002, p 187. Ryan, p 195.*) There are few bacteria for which antimicrobial susceptibility is highly predictable. However, some agents are the drug of choice because of their relative effectiveness. Among the three antibiotics that have been shown to treat legionellosis effectively (erythromycin, rifampin, and minocycline), erythromycin is clearly superior, even though in vitro studies show the organism to be susceptible to other antibiotics.

Penicillin remains the drug of choice for S. pneumoniae and the group A streptococci, although a few isolates of penicillin-resistant pneumococci have been observed. Resistance among the pneumococci is either chromosomally mediated, in which case the minimal inhibitory concentrations (MICs) are relatively low, or plasmid-mediated, which results in highly resistant bacteria. The same is generally true for H. influenzae. Until the mid-1970s, virtually all isolates of H. influenzae were susceptible to ampicillin. There has been a rapidly increasing incidence of ampicillin-resistant isolates—almost 35 to 40% in some areas of the United States. Resistance is ordinarily mediated by β-lactamase, although ampicillin-resistant, β-lactamase-negative isolates have been seen. No resistance to penicillin has been seen in group A streptococci.

Lyme disease, caused by B. burgdorferi, has been treated with penicillin, erythromycin, and tetracycline. Treatment failures have been observed. Ceftriaxone has become the drug of choice, particularly in the advanced stages of Lyme disease.

C. difficile causes toxin-mediated pseudomembranous enterocolitis as well as antibiotic-associated diarrhea. Pseudomembranous enterocolitis is normally seen during or after administration of antibiotics. One of the few agents effective against C. difficile is vancomycin. Alternatively, bacitracin can be used.

257–260. The answers are 257-a, 258-d, 259-b, 260-c. (*Brooks, pp 235–238. Levinson, pp 125–127. Murray—2002, pp 281–286. Ryan, pp 373–378.*) Some organisms originally thought to be vibrios, such as C. jejuni, have been reclassified. C. jejuni, which grows best at 42°C, has its reservoir in birds and mammals and causes gastroenteritis in humans.

V. cholerae causes cholera, which is worldwide in distribution. The three serotypes for cholera are Ogawa (AB), Inaba (AC), and Hikojima (ABC). The isolate of V. cholerae is "string-test"-positive.

V. parahaemolyticus is a halophilic marine vibrio that causes gastroenteritis in humans, primarily from ingestion of cooked seafood. It is lactose-negative and sucrose-negative.

V. vulnificus is also halophilic. It has been suggested that these halophilic vibrios do not belong in the genus *Vibrio* but in the genus *Beneckea*. *V. vulnificus* is lactose-positive and produces heat-labile, extracellular toxin. Organisms that, unlike *V. cholerae,* do not agglutinate in 0-1 antiserum were once called nonagglutinable (NAG), or noncholera (NC), vibrios. Such a classification can be confusing because *V. vulnificus,* which is an NCV, nevertheless causes severe cholera-like disease. In addition, *V. vulnificus* can produce wound infections, septicemia, meningitis, pneumonia, and keratitis.

261–264. The answers are 261-b, 262-d, 263-a, 264-e. (*Brooks, pp 246–248, 250–253. Levinson, pp 138–141. Murray—2002, pp 276–278, 305–314. Ryan, pp 401–402, 481–488.*) The organisms described in the questions all are short, ovoid, gram-negative rods. For the most part, they are nutritionally fastidious and require blood or blood products for growth. These and related organisms are unique among bacteria in that, though they have an animal reservoir, they can be transmitted to humans. Humans become infected by a variety of routes, including ingestion of contaminated animal products (*B. abortus* in cattle), direct contact with contaminated animal material or with infected animals themselves (*Y. enterocolitica* and *B. bronchiseptica* in dogs), and animal bites (*P. multocida* in many different animals). The laboratory differentiation of these microbes may be difficult and must rely on a number of parameters, including biochemical and serologic reactions, development of specific antibody response in affected persons, and epidemiologic evidence of infection.

265–267. The answers are 265-d, 266-e, 267-b. (*Brooks, pp 235, 255, 275. Levinson, pp 99, 119, 137. Murray—2002, pp 260, 285, 375. Ryan, pp 339, 373, 449.*) The medium of choice for the isolation of pathogenic Neisseriae is Thayer-Martin (TM) agar. TM agar is both a selective and an enriched medium; it contains hemoglobin, the supplement Isovitalex, and the antibiotics vancomycin, colistin, nystatin, and trimethoprim. *V. cholerae* as well as other vibrios, including *V. parahaemolyticus* and *V. alginolyticus,* are isolated best on thiosulfate citrate bile salts sucrose medium, although media such as mannitol salt agar also support the growth of vibrios. Maximal growth occurs at a pH of 8.5 to 9.5 and at 37°C incubation. Löwenstein-Jensen slants or plates, which are composed of a nutrient base and egg yolk, are used routinely for the initial isolation of mycobacteria. Small inocula of *M. tuberculosis* can also be grown in oleic acid albumin media; large inocula can be cultured on simple synthetic media.

268. The answer is b. *(Brooks, pp 183–184. Levinson, p 110. Murray—2002, pp 347–349. Ryan, pp 320–322.)* Botulism is a disease brought about by ingesting a preformed toxin. Anaerobic bacteria have grown in food, deposited the botulism toxin, and died. The toxin affects the CNS by inhibiting the release of acetylcholine at the neuronal synapse. This results in a flaccid paralysis and death by respiratory failure. At no stage of the disease will any antibiotic be able to modify or arrest the disease. Antitoxins (A, B, E) must be promptly administered, and ventilation assisted mechanically. In all other choices, antibiotics will provide a mechanism to kill or inhibit the microorganisms, bringing the infection under control.

269. The answer is d. *(Brooks, pp 292–293. Levinson, pp 157–158. Murray—2002, pp 391–393. Ryan, pp 430–431.)* Leptospirosis is a zoonosis of worldwide distribution. Human infection results from ingestion of water or food contaminated with leptospirae. Rats, mice, wild rodents, dogs, swine, and cattle excrete the organisms in urine and feces during active illness and during an asymptomatic carrier state. Drinking, swimming, bathing, or food consumption may lead to human infection. Children acquire the disease from dogs more often than do adults. Treatment can include doxycycline, ampicillin, or amoxicillin. Symptoms in humans range from fever and rash to jaundice through aseptic meningitis.

270–273. The answers are 270-e, 271-a, 272-b, 273-d. *(Brooks, p 177. Levinson, pp 23–24. Murray—2002, pp 78–81. Ryan, p 143.)* An understanding of normal, or indigenous, microflora is essential in order to appreciate the abnormal. Usually, anatomic sites contiguous to mucous membranes are not sterile and have a characteristic normal flora.

The skin flora differ as a function of location. Skin adjacent to mucous membranes may share some of the normal flora of the gastrointestinal system. Overall, the predominant bacteria on the skin surface are *S. epidermidis* and *Propionibacterium*, an anaerobic diphtheroid.

The mouth is part of the gastrointestinal tract, but its indigenous flora show some distinct differences. While anaerobes are present in large numbers, particularly in the gingival crevice, the eruption of teeth at six to nine months of age leads to colonization by organisms such as *S. mutans* and *Streptococcus sanguis*, both α-hemolytic streptococci. An edentulous person loses α-hemolytic streptococci as normal flora.

The gastrointestinal tract is sterile at birth and soon develops characteristic flora as a function of diet. In the adult, anaerobes such as *B. fragilis* and *Bifidobacterium* may outnumber coliforms and enterococci by a ratio of 1000:1. The colon contains 10^{11} to 10^{12} bacteria per gram of feces.

Soon after birth, the vagina becomes colonized by lactobacilli. As the female matures, lactobacilli may still be predominant, but anaerobic cocci, diphtheroids, and anaerobic, gram-negative rods also are found as part of the indigenous flora. Changes in the chemical or microbiologic ecology of the vagina can have marked effects on normal flora and may promote infection such as vaginitis or vaginosis.

274–277. The answers are 274-c, 275-d, 276-a, 277-e. (*Brooks, pp 192–194, 207–208. Levinson, pp 96–98, 149–150. Murray—2002, pp 229–230, 336–337. Ryan, pp 274–275, 457–459.*) *S. salivarius, S. mutans, A. israelii,* and *A. viscosus* are all part of the normal microbiota of the human mouth. Both genera are common causes of bacterial endocarditis. *S. mutans* is highly cariogenic (i.e., capable of producing dental caries), in large part because of its unique ability to synthesize a dextran bioadhesive that sticks to teeth. *S. salivarius* settles onto the mucosal epithelial surfaces of the human mouth soon after birth and is often found in the saliva. Members of the genus *Actinomyces* that are clinically significant can be differentiated by specific fluorescent antibody microscopy as well as a battery of physiologic tests, such as those assessing requirements for oxygen. *Actinomyces* organisms are opportunistic members of the normal oral microbiota. Both *A. israelii* and *A. viscosus* are pathogenic and can cause osteomyelitis in the cervicofacial region. Of the two species, *A. israelii,* which is anaerobic, is the more common causative agent of actinomycosis. *A. viscosus,* a facultative anaerobe, appears to be cariogenic.

278–284. The answers are 278-b, 279-a, 280-e, 281-d, 282-c, 283-c, 284-a. (*Brooks, pp 190–191, 244–253, 255–260. Levinson, pp 103–105, 112–113, 134–141. Murray—2002, pp 252–253, 261–265, 305–314.*) Diphtheria, a disease caused by *C. diphtheriae,* usually begins as a pharyngitis associated with pseudomembrane formation and lymphadenopathy. Grow-ing organisms lysogenic for a prophage produce a potent exotoxin that is absorbed in mucous membranes and causes remote damage to the liver, kidneys, and heart; the polypeptide toxin inhibits protein synthesis of the host cell. Although *C. diphtheriae* may infect the skin, it rarely invades the bloodstream and never actively invades deep tissue. Diphtheria toxin (DT) kills sensitive cells by blocking protein synthesis. DT is converted to an enzyme that inactivates elongation factor 2 (EF-2), which is responsible for the translocation of polypeptidyl-tRNA from the acceptor to the donor site on the eukaryotic ribosome. The reaction is as follows:

$$NAD + EF\text{-}2 = ADP\text{-}ribosyl - EF\text{-}2 + nicotinamide + H^+$$

B. pertussis and *B. parapertussis* are similar and may be isolated together from a clinical specimen. However, *B. parapertussis* does not produce per-tussis toxin. Pertussis toxin, like many bacterial toxins, has two subunits: A and B. Subunit A is an active enzyme, and B promotes binding of the toxin to host cells.

F. tularensis is a short, gram-negative organism that is markedly pleo-morphic; it is nonmotile and cannot form spores. It has a rigid growth requirement for cysteine. Human tularemia usually is acquired from direct contact with tissues of infected rabbits but also can be transmitted by the bites of flies and ticks. *F. tularensis* causes a variety of clinical syndromes, including ulceroglandular, oculoglandular, pneumonic, and typhoidal forms of tularemia.

The pathogenesis of infection with *E. coli* is a complex interrelation of many events and properties. *E. coli* may serve as a model for other members of the Enterobacteriaceae. Some strains of *E. coli* are enteroinvasive (EIEC), some enterotoxic (ETEC), some enterohemorrhagic (EHEC), and others enteropathogenic (EPEC). At the present time, there is little clinical signif-icance in routinely discriminating the various types, with the possible exceptions of the ETEC and the *E. coli* 0157/H7 that are hemorrhagic. *E. coli* 0157/H7 secretes a toxin called *verotoxin*. The toxin is very active in a Vero cell line. More correctly, the toxin(s) should be called *Shiga-like*.

Streptococcal infection usually is accompanied by an elevated titer of antibody to some of the enzymes produced by the organism. Among the anti-genic substances elaborated by group A β-hemolytic streptococci are erythrogenic toxin, streptodornase (streptococcal DNase), hyaluronidase, and streptolysin O (a hemolysin). Streptolysin S is a nonantigenic hemolysin. Specifically, erythrogenic toxin causes the characteristic rash of scarlet fever.

Many factors play a role in the pathogenesis of *N. meningitidis*. A capsule containing N-acetylneuraminic acid is peculiar to *Neisseria* and *E. coli* K1. Fresh isolates carry pili on their surfaces, which function in adhesion. *Neisseria* has a variety of membrane proteins, and their role in pathogenesis can only be speculated upon at this time. The lipopolysaccharide (LPS) of *Neisseria*, more correctly called lipooligosaccharide (LOS), is the endotoxic component of the cell.

There are no known toxins, hemolysins, or cell-wall constituents known to play a role in the pathogenesis of disease by *Brucella*. Rather, the ability of the organisms to survive within the host phagocyte and to inhibit neutrophil degranulation is a major disease-causing factor. In infectious abortion of cattle caused by *Brucella*, the tropism for placenta and the chorion is a function of the presence of erythritol in allantoic and amniotic fluid.

285–289.   The answers are 285-a, 286-b, 287-c, 288-b, 289-c. *(Ryan, pp 851–855.)* "Atypical pneumonia" is an old classification used for respiratory disease that is not lobar and is not "typical." That is, it does not include pneumonia caused by pneumococcus, *Klebsiella, Haemophilus,* or β-hemolytic streptococci that results in a typical lobular infiltrate. In recent years, the atypical pneumonias have become much more frequent than pneumococcal pneumonia. They are characterized by a slower onset with headache, joint pain, fever, and signs of an acute upper respiratory infection. There are usually no signs of acute respiratory distress, but patients report malaise and fatigue. The most common cause of atypical pneumonia is *M. pneumoniae.* A quick test for *M. pneumoniae* infection is cold agglutinins. The test may lack both sensitivity and specificity, but it is rapid and readily available compared with culture of *M. pneumoniae* or specific antibody formation.

Particularly in the winter months, influenza must be ruled out. In the early stages of an epidemic, viral isolation in primary monkey cells is used. However, as the epidemic proceeds, diagnosis is usually made clinically or by an increase in antibody titer.

In certain age groups (men over 55 years old), Legionnaires' disease must be ruled out. While direct microscopy, culture, and serology are available, the detection of *Legionella* antigen in respiratory secretions is the most sensitive test available.

C. pneumoniae may also cause respiratory infection particularly in, but not limited to, children. Diagnosis is best made by growing these energy-defective bacteria in tissue culture such as HeLa cells. Serology is usually not helpful.

During the winter months, *Bordetella* infection may be quite prevalent, particularly in those patients whose immunizations are not current. Adult *Bordetella* infection may not present with typical whooping cough symptoms and must be differentiated from other forms of acute bronchitis by culture on specific media or direct fluorescent microscopy.

Rickettsiae, Chlamydiae, and Mycoplasmas

Questions

DIRECTIONS: Each question below contains four or more suggested responses. Select the **one best** response to each question.

290. Which of the following describes the difference between mycoplasmas and chlamydiae?

a. Able to cause disease in humans
b. Able to cause urinary tract infection
c. Able to grow on artificial cell-free media
d. Able to stain well with Gram stain
e. Susceptible to penicillin

291. A 39-year-old man presented with sudden, influenza-like symptoms. He stated that he worked in a slaughterhouse, and several of his coworkers had similar symptoms. Early stages of pneumonia were detected. A rickettsial etiology was suspected. Which of the following characterizes Q fever?

a. Has an incubation period of four to six weeks
b. Is an acute febrile illness caused by *Coxiella burnetii*
c. Is an illness confined to the upper respiratory tract
d. Is most commonly found in tropical regions
e. Is transmitted by the bite of an arthropod

292. Which of the following characterizes rickettsiae, which include the spotted fevers, Q fever, typhus, and scrub typhus?

a. Easily stained (gram-negative) with a Gram stain
b. Maintained in nature, with humans as the mammalian reservoir
c. Obligate intracellular parasites
d. Stable outside the host cell
e. The cause of infections in which a rash is always present

293. A man with chills, fever, and headache is thought to have "atypical" pneumonia. History reveals that he raises chickens and that approximately two weeks ago he lost a large number of them to an undiagnosed disease. Which of the following is the most likely diagnosis of this man's condition?

a. Anthrax
b. Leptospirosis
c. Ornithosis
d. Relapsing fever
e. Q fever

294. An ill patient denied being bitten by insects. However, he had spent some time in a milking barn and indicated that it was dusty. Of the following rickettsial diseases, which one has he most likely contracted?

a. Brill-Zinsser disease
b. Q fever
c. Rickettsialpox
d. Rocky Mountain spotted fever (RMSF)
e. Scrub typhus

295. A 23-year-old college senior presented to the student health clinic with symptoms of a suspected sexually transmitted disease (STD). *Neisseria* and *Chlamydia* agents were ruled out. Which of the following organisms was the most likely cause of his nongonococcal urethritis (NGU)?

a. *Mycoplasma fermentans*
b. *Mycoplasma hominis*
c. *Mycoplasma mycoides*
d. *Mycoplasma pneumoniae*
e. *Ureaplasma urealyticum*

296. A young man, home on leave from the military, went camping in the woods to detect deer movement for future hunting. Ten days later, he developed fever, malaise, and myalgia. Leukopenia and thromboceptopenia were observed, as well as several tick bites. Which of the following statements best describes human monocytic ehrlichiosis (HME)?

a. Clinical diagnosis is based on the presence of erythema migrans (EM)
b. Diagnosis is usually made serologically but morulae may be seen in the cytoplasm of monocytes
c. It is a fatal disease transmitted by the bite of a dog
d. Symptoms include vomiting and paralysis
e. The HME agent grows on artificial media

297. Lymphogranuloma venereum (LGV) is a venereal disease caused by serotype L1, L2, or L3 of *Chlamydia trachomatis*. The differential diagnosis should include which of the following?

a. Babesiosis
b. Chancroid
c. Mononucleosis
d. Psittacosis
e. Shingles

298. A forest worker experienced a sudden onset of fever, headache, myalgias, and prostration. A mascular rash developed several days later, with it appearing first on the hands and feet before moving onto his trunk. Rocky Mountain spotted fever was diagnosed. Which treatment is utilized for this disease?

a. Amphoteracin B
b. Cephalosporin
c. Erythromycin
d. Sulfonamides
e. Tetracycline

299. *C. trachomatis* can be distinguished from *Chlamydia psittaci* by which of the following criteria?

a. *C. psittaci* forms inclusions that contain glycogen
b. *C. psittaci* is an obligate prokaryotic parasite
c. *C. trachomatis* can be stained with Giemsa
d. *C. trachomatis* has a different lipopolysaccharide antigen
e. *C. trachomatis* is sensitive to sulfonamides

300. Chlamydiae have an unusual three-stage cycle of development. Which of the following is the correct sequence of these events?

a. Development of an initial body, synthesis of elementary body progeny, penetration of the host cell
b. Penetration of the host cell, development of an initial body, synthesis of elementary body progeny
c. Penetration of the host cell, synthesis of elementary body progeny, development of an initial body
d. Synthesis of elementary body progeny, development of an initial body, penetration of the host cell
e. Synthesis of elementary body progeny, penetration of the host cell, development of an initial body

301. Young children in a small Egyptian village had eye infections that presented with lacrimation, discharge, and conjunctival hyperemia. Scarring of the conjunctiva and noticeable loss of vision occurred in some. Which of the following statements would describe the etiologic agent causing these infections and relative treatment?

a. The organisms are gram-positive and treatable with penicillin
b. The organisms have no cell wall and will only respond to tetracycline
c. The organisms are gram-negative, and prophylactic use of tetracyclines can prevent infections
d. Gram stains of conjunctival scrapings are useful diagnostic tests to justify treatment with sulfonamides
e. The organisms are isolated on blood agar plates and respond to cell-wall inhibiting antibiotics

302. Human granulocytic ehrlichiosis (HGE) is a disease transmitted to humans by the bite of a tick, *Ixodes scapularis*. Which of the following statements about HGE is most correct?

a. Clinical diagnosis is based on the presence of erythema migrans
b. HGE is caused by *Ehrlichia chaffeensis*
c. HGE is a self-limiting disease
d. HGE is characterized by an acute onset of fever, severe headache, and influenza-like symptoms
e. The causative organism can be grown on ordinary laboratory media

303. The "spotted fever" group of rickettsial diseases is caused by a variety of rickettsial species. While not critical for treatment of disease, the speciation of these organisms is essential for epidemiologic studies. Of the following rickettsiae, which one is found in the United States and is a member of the spotted fever group?

a. *Rickettsia akari*
b. *Rickettsia australis*
c. *Rickettsia conorii*
d. *Rickettsia prowazekii*
e. *Rickettsia sibirica*

304. A 36-year-old man presented at his physician's office complaining of fever and headache. On examination, he had leukopenia and increased liver enzymes, and inclusion bodies were seen in his monocytes. History revealed that he was an outdoorsman and remembered removing a tick from his leg. Which of the following diseases most likely caused the symptoms described?

a. Ehrlichiosis
b. Lyme disease
c. Q fever
d. Rocky Mountain spotted fever
e. Tularemia

305. Typhus, spotted fever, and scrub typhus share which of the following manifestations of disease?

a. Arthritis
b. Common vector
c. Fever and rash
d. Short incubation period (<48 h)
e. Similar geographic distribution

306. *C. trachomatis* is a well-known cause of venereal disease. This organism is also implicated in which of the following?

a. Classic trachoma infection
b. Middle-ear infection in young children
c. Perinatal retinitis
d. Sexually transmitted cardiac disease in adults
e. Urinary tract infection in children

307. A homosexual male presented to his physician with bilateral inguinal buboes (lymph nodes), one of which seemed ready to rupture. He recalled having two small, painless genital lesions that healed rapidly. The etiologic agent was isolated using McCoy cells. Which one of the following statements best characterizes lymphogranuloma venereum (LGV)?

a. It is most common in temperate regions
b. In the United States, it is more common among women
c. The causative agent is *C. trachomatis*
d. The disease (LGV) does not become chronic
e. Penicillin is effective in early treatment

308. Dozens of political refugees fleeing from active warfare and living in a dense forest environment with crowded, unsanitary conditions experienced nonspecific symptoms, followed by high fever and severe headache, along with chills, myalgia, and arthralgia. All had body lice. Improved living conditions in a refugee camp and treatment with tetracycline brought resolution to most individuals. Which of the following statements describes the etiological agent responsible for their infection?

a. The disease was caused by an organism with no cell walls
b. The disease was caused by a viral agent
c. The disease was derived from rodents living in the forest area
d. Reoccurance of milder disease may occur in later years
e. The disease was caused by a tick vector

309. Chlamydiae are small, gram-negative rods once thought to be viruses. Which of the following best characterizes chlamydiae as distinct from viruses?

a. Cannot visualize with light microscope
b. Independent synthesis of proteins
c. Intracellular reproduction
d. Susceptibility to antimicrobial agents
e. Synthesis of ATP

310. *Chlamydia pneumoniae,* sometimes known as *Chlamydia* "TWAR," is the most recent *Chlamydia* species to be associated with human disease. Which one of the following statements best describes *C. pneumoniae?*

a. *C. pneumoniae* has been associated with myocardial infarction
b. *C. pneumoniae* infections are generally severe
c. *C. pneumoniae* infections are uncommon—up to 10% of adults may show specific antibody
d. Infections with *C. pneumoniae* usually arise from bacterial overgrowth in the colon
e. Nonpsittacine birds are reservoirs of *C. pneumoniae*

Item 311–314

Members of the genus of *Mycoplasma* have a variety of clinical and epidemiological features.

311. Which one of the following organisms causes primary atypical pneumonia in humans?

a. *M. fermentans*
b. *M. hominis*
c. *M. pneumoniae*
d. *Mycoplasma orale*
e. *U. urealyticum*

312. Which one of the following organisms is associated with nongonococcal urethritis in humans?

a. *M. fermentans*
b. *M. hominis*
c. *M. pneumoniae*
d. *M. orale*
e. *U. urealyticum*

313. Which one of the following organisms normally inhabits the healthy human oral cavity?

a. *M. fermentans*
b. *M. hominis*
c. *M. pneumoniae*
d. *M. orale*
e. *U. urealyticum*

314. Which one of the following organisms normally inhabits the female genital tract but may cause acute respiratory illness?

a. *M. fermentans*
b. *M. hominis*
c. *M. pneumoniae*
d. *M. orale*
e. *U. urealyticum*

Item 315–319

The following group of organisms is characterized as difficult to cultivate, with some interesting molecular and physiologic similarities.

Bartonella (Rochalimaea) henselae
C. trachomatis
C. burnetii
E. chaffeensis
Rickettsia rickettsii

315. Which of the following is the causative agent of lymphogranuloma venereum?

a. *B. (Rochalimaea) henselae*
b. *C. trachomatis*
c. *C. burnetii*
d. *E. chaffeensis*
e. *R. rickettsii*

316. Which one of the following is transmitted by the bite of a hard *Ixodes* tick?

a. *B. (Rochalimaea) henselae*
b. *C. trachomatis*
c. *C. burnetii*
d. *E. chaffeensis*
e. *R. rickettsii*

317. Which of the following microorganisms is the causative agent of cat-scratch disease?

a. *B. (Rochalimaea) henselae*
b. *C. trachomatis*
c. *C. burnetii*
d. *E. chaffeensis*
e. *R. rickettsii*

318. Which of the following is a gram-negative rickettsia with tropism for mononuclear cells and causes Q fever?

a. *B. (Rochalimaea) henselae*
b. *C. trachomatis*
c. *C. burnetii*
d. *E. chaffeensis*
e. *R. rickettsii*

319. Which of the following is the causative agent of Rocky Mountain spotted fever?

a. *B. (Rochalimaea) henselae*
b. *C. trachomatis*
c. *C. burnetii*
d. *E. chaffeensis*
e. *R. rickettsii*

Rickettsiae, Chlamydiae, and Mycoplasmas

Answers

290. The answer is c. (*Brooks, pp 295, 306. Levinson, pp 151, 159. Murray—2002, pp 395, 412. Ryan, pp 409, 463.*) Mycoplasmas lack a rigid cell wall and are bound by a triple-layer unit membrane. For this reason, they are completely resistant to the action of penicillins. Unlike the chlamydiae, they can replicate in cell-free media.

291. The answer is b. (*Brooks, p 302. Levinson, p 163. Murray—2002, pp 409–410. Ryan, p 477.*) Q fever is an acute, flulike illness caused by *C. burnetii*. It is the one rickettsial disease not transmitted by the bite of a tick. *C. burnetii* is found in high concentrations in the urine, feces, and placental tissue/amniotic fluid of cattle, goats, and sheep. Transmission to humans is by aerosol inhalation of those specimens.

292. The answer is c. (*Brooks, p 301. Levinson, p 162. Murray—2002, p 401. Ryan, pp 472–473.*) Rickettsiae are obligate intracellular parasites that depend on host cells for their phosphorylated energy compounds. The significant rickettsial diseases in North America include Rocky Mountain spotted fever (*R. rickettsii*), Q fever (*C. burnetii*), and typhus (*R. prowazekii, Rickettsia typhi*). Laboratory diagnosis of rickettsial disease is based on serologic analysis rather than isolation of the organism.

293. The answer is c. (*Brooks, pp 313–314. Levinson, p 159. Murray—2002, pp 419–420. Ryan, p 469.*) Ornithosis (psittacosis) is caused by *C. psittaci*. Humans usually contract the disease from infected birds kept as pets or from infected poultry, including poultry in dressing plants. Although ornithosis may be asymptomatic in humans, severe pneumonia can develop. Fortunately, the disease is cured easily with tetracycline.

294. The answer is b. (*Brooks, p 302. Levinson, p 163. Murray—2002, pp 409–410. Ryan, p 477.*) Most rickettsial diseases are transmitted to humans by way of arthropod vectors. The only exception is Q fever, which is caused by *C. burnetii*. This organism is transmitted by inhalation of contaminated dust and aerosols or by ingestion of contaminated milk.

295. The answer is e. *(Brooks, p 298. Levinson, p 152. Murray—2002, p 397. Ryan, p 413.)* *U. urealyticum* has been associated with NGU as well as infertility. *M. pneumoniae* is the etiologic agent of primary atypical pneumonia. *M. hominis*, although isolated from up to 30% of patients with NGU, has yet to be implicated as a cause of that disease. *M. fermentans* has on rare occasions been isolated from the oropharynx and genital tract. *M. mycoides* causes bovine pleuropneumonia.

296. The answer is b. *(Brooks, pp 304–305. Levinson, p 167. Murray— 2002, pp 407–408. Ryan, p 478.)* HME, caused by the bite of the tick *Amblyomma americanum* infected with *E. chaffeensis*, causes an illness not unlike RMSF, except a rash usually does not occur. Diagnosis is usually made serologically, and treatment of choice is tetracycline. Symptoms include high fever, severe headache, and myalgias.

297. The answer is b. *(Brooks, p 311. Levinson, p 161. Murray—2002, pp 415–416. Ryan, pp 466–467.)* The differential diagnosis of LGV includes syphilis, genital herpes, and chancroid. Several clinical tests can be used to rule out syphilis and genital herpes. These include a positive dark-field examination as well as positive serologic findings for syphilis and the demonstration of herpes simplex virus by cytology or culture. *Haemophilus ducreyi* can usually be isolated from the ulcer in chancroid.

298. The answer is e. *(Brooks, pp 302–303. Levinson, p 164. Murray— 2002, p 401. Ryan, p 475.)* Tetracyclines and chloromphenicol are effective, provided treatment is started early. Those should be given orally daily and continued for several days after the rash subsides. IV dosage can be used in severely ill patients. Sulfonamides enhance the disease and are contraindicated. The other antibiotics are ineffective. Antibiotics only suppress the bacteria's growth, and the patient's immune system must eradicate them.

299. The answer is e. *(Brooks, p 308. Levinson, p 161. Murray—2002, p 419. Ryan, p 463.)* The chlamydiae are obligate prokaryotic parasites of eukaryotic cells. For many years, they were considered to be viruses but are now considered to be bacteria. The two species, *C. trachomatis* and

C. psittaci, can be distinguished by two criteria: the susceptibility of C. trachomatis to sulfonamides and its ability to form inclusions containing glycogen.

300. The answer is b. (Brooks, p 306. Levinson, p 160. Murray—2002, p 414. Ryan, p 465.) The developmental cycle of chlamydiae begins with the elementary body attaching to and then penetrating the host cell. The elementary body, now in a vacuole bounded by host-cell membrane, becomes an initial body. Within about 12 hours, the initial body has divided to form many small elementary particles encased within an inclusion body in the cytoplasm; these progeny are liberated by host-cell rupture.

301. The answer is c. (Brooks, pp 306–308. Levinson, pp 159–161. Murray—2002, pp 414–416. Ryan, pp 464–466.) C. trachomatis serovars A, B, Ba, and C are responsible for endemic trachoma. While diagnosis is usually dependent upon observation of intracellular inclusions with a glycogen matrix in which elementary bodies are embedded, Gram stain preparations are not useful diagnostic tools. The cell wall most closely resembles a gram high lipid content and may stain gram-negative or variable. A single monthly dose of doxycycline can result in significant clinical improvement and be preventative.

302. The answer is d. (Brooks, pp 304–305. Levinson, p 158. Murray—2002, p 408. Ryan, p 478.) HGE is caused by the bite of I. scapularis infected with either Ehrlichia phagocytophilia or Ehrlichia ewingii. A rash rarely occurs and erythema migrans (EM) does not occur, but the symptoms (fever, chills, headache, myalgia, nausea, vomiting, anorexia, and weight loss) are similar to those seen in RMSF. Serological tests show that subclinical ehrlichiosis occurs frequently.

303. The answer is a. (Brooks, p 301. Levinson, p 163. Murray—2002, p 402. Ryan, p 473.) The primary cause of Rocky Mountain spotted fever (RMSF) is R. rickettsii, although rickettsialpox is caused by R. akari, the only other member of the spotted fever group that resides in the United States. R. sibirica is responsible for tick typhus in China; R. australis causes typhus in Australia, as the name signifies; and R. conorii causes European and African rickettsioses. R. prowazekii is not a member of the spotted fever group; it causes epidemic typhus.

304. The answer is a. (*Brooks, pp 304, 305. Levinson, p 167. Murray—2002, pp 407–408. Ryan, p 478.*) All the listed diseases except Q fever are tick-borne. The rickettsia *C. burnetii* causes Q fever, and humans are usually infected by aerosol of a sporelike form shed in milk, urine, feces, or placenta of infected sheep, cattle, or goats. Lyme disease is caused by a spirochete, *Borrelia burgdorferi,* and produces the characteristic lesion erythema chronicum migrans (ECM). The etiologic agent of Rocky Mountain spotted fever is *R. rickettsia.* It usually produces a rash that begins in the extremities and then involves the trunk. Two human forms of ehrlichiosis can occur: human monocytic ehrlichiosis (HME), caused by *E. chaffeensis,* and human granulocytic ehrlichiosis (HGE), caused by an as yet unnamed *Ehrlichia.* Ehrlichiosis was previously recognized only as a veterinary pathogen. HME infection is transmitted by the brown dog tick and *A. americanum.* HGE infection is transmitted by *I. scapularis,* the same tick that transmits Lyme disease. Both infections cause fever and leukopenia. A rash rarely occurs. *E. chaffeensis* infects monocytes, and HGE infects granulocytes; both organisms produce inclusion bodies called *morulae. Francisella tularensis* is a small, gram-negative, nonmotile coccobacillus. Humans most commonly acquire the organism after contact with the tissues or body fluid of an infected mammal or the bite of an infected tick.

305. The answer is c. (*Brooks, p 301. Levinson, pp 162–164. Murray—2002, p 404. Ryan, pp 473–475.*) Typhus, spotted fever, and scrub typhus are all caused by rickettsiae (*R. prowazekii, R. rickettsii,* and *Rickettsia tsutsugamushi,* respectively). Clinically, the diseases have several similarities. Each has an incubation period of one to two weeks, followed by a febrile period, which usually includes a rash. During the febrile period, rickettsiae can be found in the patient's blood and there is disseminated focal vasculitis of small blood vessels. The geographic area associated with these diseases is usually different. Scrub typhus is usually found in Japan, Southeast Asia, and the Pacific, while spotted fever is usually found in the Western hemisphere. Typhus has a worldwide incidence.

306. The answer is a. (*Brooks, pp 308–309. Levinson, p 160. Murray—2002, p 413. Ryan, p 464.*) Trachoma has been the greatest single cause of blindness in the world. *C. trachomatis* is the most common cause of sexually transmitted disease in the United States and is also responsible for the majority of cases of infant conjunctivitis and infant pneumonia.

307. The answer is c. (*Brooks, pp 309–310. Levinson, pp 160–161. Murray—2002, pp 416–417. Ryan, pp 466–468.*) LGV is a sexually transmitted disease caused by *C. trachomatis* of immunotypes L1, L2, and L3. It is more commonly found in tropical climates. In the United States, the sex ratio is reported to be 3.4 males to 1 female. Tetracycline has been successful in treating this disease in the early stages; however, late stages usually require surgery.

308. The answer is d. (*Brooks, pp 303–304. Levinson, pp 163–164. Murray—2002, pp 405–406. Ryan, pp 475–476.*) The disease described is epidemic typhus or louse-borne typhus. It is caused by *R. prowazekii* and is spread by the human body louse, *Pediculus humanus*. Lice obviously occur most readily in unsanitary conditions brought on by war or natural disasters, where normal healthy living conditions are unavailable. Rickettsial diseases respond to tetracycline treatment and vector control. The organisms replicate in endothelial cells, resulting in vasculitis. Recrudescent disease (recurrence in later years) has been demonstrated in people exposed to epidemic typhus during World War II. This form of disease is generally milder, and convalescence is shorter.

309. The answer is b. (*Brooks, pp 306–307. Levinson, p 159. Murray—2002, p 412. Ryan, pp 463–464.*) Although both chlamydiae and viruses are obligate, intracellular parasites and depend on the host cell for ATP and phosphorylated intermediates, they differ in many respects. Unlike viruses, chlamydiae synthesize proteins and reproduce by fission. Chlamydiae are readily seen under the light microscope and possess bacteria-like cell walls.

310. The answer is a. (*Brooks, pp 312–313. Levinson, p 161. Murray—2002, pp 418–419. Ryan, p 470.*) A distinct group of chlamydiae, first designated "TWAR," has been given the name *C. pneumoniae*. The strain was first isolated in Taiwan and usually causes mild acute respiratory disease. *C. psittaci* causes a respiratory syndrome and is associated with avian contact. *C. pneumoniae* has no avian vector. Recent evidence suggests that *C. pneumoniae* may be involved in cardiac disease, possibly as part of an autoimmune phenomenon. This organism has recently had a genus name change to *Chlamydophila*.

311–314. The answers are 311-c, 312-e, 313-d, 314-b. (*Brooks, pp 295–298. Levinson, pp 151–152. Murray—2002, pp 395–399. Ryan,* *pp 409–412.*) Members of the mycoplasma group that are pathogenic for humans include *M. pneumoniae* and *U. urealyticum. M. pneumoniae* is best known as the causative agent of primary atypical pneumonia (PAP), which may be confused clinically with influenza or legionellosis. It also is associated with arthritis, pericarditis, aseptic meningitis, and the Guillain-Barré syndrome. *M. pneumoniae* can be cultivated on special media and identified by immunofluorescence staining and "fried egg" colonies on agar.

U. urealyticum (once called *tiny,* or *T, strain*) has been implicated in cases of nongonococcal urethritis. As the name implies, this organism is able to split urea, a fact of diagnostic significance. *U. urealyticum* is part of the normal flora of the genitourinary tract, particularly in women.

Both *M. orale* and *Mycoplasma salivarium* are inhabitants of the normal human oral cavity. These species are commensals and do not play a role in disease.

The only other species of *Mycoplasma* associated with human disease is *M. hominis.* A normal inhabitant of the genital tract of women, this organism has been demonstrated to produce an acute respiratory illness that is associated with sore throat and tonsillar exudate, but not with fever.

M. fermentans is an animal isolate.

315–319. The answers are 315-b, 316-d, 317-a, 318-c, 319-e.
(*Brooks, pp 273, 301, 305, 306–313. Levinson, pp 159–161, 162–164, 166–167. Murray—2002, pp 329–330, 401–409, 412–414. Ryan, pp 463–470, 471–479.*) Rickettsiae are small bacteria that are obligate, intracellular parasites. Most but not all rickettsiae are transmitted to humans by arthropods. *Coxiella* is transmitted through the respiratory tract rather than through the skin, and *B. henselae* from animal scratches. *Coxiella* may cause chronic endocarditis that is not very responsive to either antimicrobial therapy or valve replacement. *B. henselae* is a fastidious, gram-negative rod that causes bacillary angiomatosis, a disease that forms dermal or subcutaneous nodules. The role of *B. henselae* in cat-scratch disease has recently been recognized. Molecular taxonomic studies have indicated that the causative organism is more closely related to *Bartonella* than to *Rochalimaea,* hence the name change.

Ehrlichia is an obligate, intracellular parasite that resembles rickettsia. *E. chaffeensis* has been linked to human ehrlichiosis, although this infection is primarily seen in animals. The majority of patients with this disease report exposure to ticks. It is thought that *I. scapularis* carries *Ehrlichia,* although the Lone Star tick, *A. americanum,* may also transmit the disease.

Chlamydiae are gram-negative bacteria that are obligate, intracellular parasites. They are divided into three species: *C. trachomatis, C. pneumoniae,* and *C. psittaci.* Chlamydiae have a unique developmental cycle. The infectious particle is the elementary body. Once inside the cell, the elementary body undergoes reorganization to form a reticulate body. After several replications, the reticulate bodies differentiate into elementary bodies, are released from the host cell, and become available to infect other cells. Three of the 15 serovars of *C. trachomatis* (L1, L2, L3) are known to cause lymphogranuloma venereum (LGV), a sexually transmitted disease. *C. trachomatis* is a leading cause of sexually transmitted disease in the United States. It is insidious because so many early infections are asymptomatic, particularly in women.

Rocky Mountain spotted fever is a spotted fever caused by *R. rickettsii* and is characterized by acute onset of fever, severe headache, and myalgias. The rash occurs two to six days later, first in the hands and feet, and then moves to the trunk. Diagnosis must be made on clinical presentations, and therapy instituted immediately. Laboratory diagnosis is made on a rising antibody titer (delayed). Untreated disease can be fatal.

Mycology

Questions

DIRECTIONS: Each question below contains four or more suggested responses. Select the **one best** response to each question.

320. Infected tissues demonstrating budding fungal cells are seen in which of the following?

a. Aspergillosis, mucormycosis, and mycetoma
b. Blastomycosis, paracoccidioides, and dermatophytosis
c. Candidiasis, cryptococcosis, and sporotrichosis
d. Coccidioidomycosis, chromomycosis, and aspergillosis
e. Tinea versicolor, tinea nigra, and candidiasis

321. A 62-year-old white male was admitted to the hospital complaining of shortness of breath. His medical history indicated he had smoked one pack of cigarettes per day for the past 40 years. Recently, he has been on immunosuppressive therapy for severe arthritis. A biopsy specimen of the lung was obtained, and septate hyphae that formed V-shaped branches were observed. Culture on agar showed conidia with spores in radiating columns (see photo). Which of the following is most likely consistent with these diagnostic findings?

a. Aspergillosis
b. Emphysema
c. Lung cancer
d. *Pneumocystis carinii* pneumonia
e. Viral pneumonia
f. Zygomycosis

x1000

Aspergillus fumigatus. Phialides form on top of swollen vesicle at the end of a long conidiophore. Terminal conidium is oldest. Mature conidia have rough walls. (*Reproduced, with permission, from Brooks GF et al. Jawetz's Medical Microbiology, 22e. New York: McGraw-Hill, 2001, 534.*)

322. The object designated by the arrow in the following photomicrograph is which one of the following?

a. An encapsulated yeast
b. A hyphal strand
c. A macroconidium
d. A spherule
e. A thick-walled spore

323. A 6-year-old girl presented to the clinic with scaly patches on the scalp. Primary smears and culture of the skin and hair were negative. A few weeks later, she returned and was found to have inflammatory lesions. The hair fluoresced under Wood's light and primary smears of skin and hair contained septate hyphae. On speaking with the parents, it was discovered that there were several pets in the household. Which of the following is the most likely agent?

a. *Epidermophyton floccosum*
b. *Microsporum audouinii*
c. *Microsporum canis*
d. *Trichophyton rubrum*
e. *Trichophyton tonsurans*

324. A patient with AIDS has a persistent cough and has shown progressive behavioral changes in the past few weeks after eating an undercooked hamburger. A cerebrospinal fluid (CSF) sample is collected and an encapsulated, yeastlike organism is observed. Based only on these observations, what is the most likely organism?

a. *Candida*
b. *Cryptococcus*
c. *Cryptosporidium*
d. *Pneumocystis*
e. *Toxoplasma*

325. A chronically ill, young, white male was unable to work due to his frequent illnesses. He spent most of his time raising and training pigeons. He developed a mild pulmonary infection and eventually presented with headache, mental status changes, and fever. A clinical diagnosis of meningitis was confirmed with a latex agglutination test on CSF for the capsular polysaccharide of the organism. What is the most likely causative agent?

a. *Aspergillus fumigatus*
b. *Candida albicans*
c. *Cryptococcus neoformans*
d. *Histoplasma capsulatum*
e. *Paracoccidioides brasiliensis*

326. A section of tissue from the foot of a person assumed to have eumycotic mycetoma shows a white, lobulated granule composed of fungal hyphae. In the United States, the most common etiologic agent of this condition is a species of which of the following?

a. *Acremonium*
b. *Actinomyces*
c. *Madurella*
d. *Nocardia*
e. *Pseudallescheria*

327. The formation of granulomas is seen in major systemic fungal infections. Which of the following groups of fungi is most likely to cause granulomas?

a. *Aspergillus, Coccidioides, Cryptococcus*
b. *Epidermophyton, Blastomyces, Trichophyton*
c. *Cladosporium, Aspergillus, Microsporum*
d. *Coccidioides, Blastomyces, Histoplasma*
e. *Mucor, Candida, Malassezia*

328. Infection with *Sporothrix schenckii* (formerly *Sporotrichum schenckii*) is an occupational hazard for gardeners. The portal of entry for this organism is via which of the following routes?

a. Lymphatic system
b. Mouth
c. Mucous membranes
d. Respiratory tract
e. Skin

329. There are three genera of dermatophytes: *Epidermophyton, Microsporum,* and *Trichophyton.* Which of the following statements characterizes the infections caused by these organisms, as shown in the figure below (dermatophytoses)?

(Courtesy of MG Rinaldi, San Antonio, TX)

a. Characterized by aflatoxin-induced hallucinations
b. Confined to keratinized tissues
c. Easily treatable with penicillin
d. Marked by alveolar irritation
e. Rarely associated with chronic lesions

330. A 57-year-old obese white female was referred to your clinic due to a sore throat characterized by a white pseudomembranous lesion of epithelial cells and organisms. The patient's history revealed type 1 diabetes mellitus and recent penicillin use for a severe bacterial infection in her right foot. *C. albicans* was recognized in microscopic examination of infected tissues by the presence of which of the following?

a. Abundance of septate rhizoids
b. Asci containing two to eight ascospores
c. Metachromatic granules
d. Spherules containing endospores
e. Yeasts and pseudohyphae

331. The mechanism of mucosal invasion by *C. albicans* is at least partially understood. Which one of the following modifications in the structure or function of this yeast would be most likely to affect its invasive ability?

a. Loss of ability to produce ethanol from glucose
b. Loss of ability to produce germ tubes or hyphae
c. Loss of ability to produce a polysaccharide capsule
d. Reduced ability to grow at 37°C
e. Replacement of mannans in the cell wall with glucan

332. You have been designated as coordinator of construction of a bone marrow transplant unit (BMTU). There will be extensive removal of walls and floors in order to install the laminar flow rooms required for a BMTU. From the standpoint of frequency and lethality, which one of the following fungi should be your biggest concern?

a. *Aspergillus*
b. *Blastomyces*
c. *Candida*
d. *Cryptococcus*
e. *Wangiella*

333. *H. capsulatum,* a dimorphic fungus, is found in soil heavily contaminated with bird droppings. Which of the following statements best describes the presence of the organism in tissue biopsies?

a. Arthrospores
b. Oval budding yeasts inside macrophages
c. Single-cell yeasts with pseudohyphae
d. Spherules containing endospores
e. Yeasts with broad-based bud

334. Which of the following best describes an infection with *Coccidioides immitis?*

a. A negative complement-fixing (CF) antibody test
b. Clavate macroconidia
c. "Fungus ball" formation
d. Inhaled arthrospores form thick-walled spherules filled with endospores
e. Thrush

335. Inhalation of fungal spores can cause primary lung infections. Of the following organisms, which one is most likely to be associated with this mode of transmission?

a. *C. albicans*
b. *Candida tropicalis*
c. *C. immitis*
d. *S. schenckii*
e. *T. tonsurans*

336. An immunocompromised patient is suspected of having an infection with *A. fumigatus.* Which of the following clinical conditions is most likely to occur?

a. Invasive infection causing thrombosis and infarction
b. Superficial rash
c. Thrush
d. Urinary tract infection
e. Wound infection

337. A 25-year-old pregnant woman, living in the San Joaquin Valley (California) experienced an influenza-like illness with fever and cough. She was diagnosed with *Coccidioides* infection that disseminated from her lungs to other organs while in the third trimester of pregnancy. Patients who have disseminated coccidioidomycosis usually demonstrate which one of the following?

a. Absence of complement-fixing (CF) antibodies
b. A negative coccidioidin skin test and a rising CF titer
c. A negative coccidioidin skin test and a stable CF titer
d. A positive skin test and a mildly elevated CF titer
e. Lack of immunity to reinfection

Questions 338–341

338. *C. albicans* (shown below) is best described by which of the following statements?

(Courtesy of MG Rinaldi, San Antonio, TX)

a. Round, black sporangia filled with endospores; sporangia unbranched, rising from a runner called a stolon
b. Single-tipped sporangiophores; no rhizoids or stolons; nonseptate hyphae, which show branching
c. Widespread in environment; conidia may be inhaled; microscopic appearance in specimen reveals dichotomous branching and septate hyphae
d. Yeast forms with budding blastoconidia often showing pseudohyphae; positive germ tube test; chlamydospores present

339. *Aspergillus* is best described by which of the following statements?

a. Round, black sporangia filled with endospores; sporangia unbranched, rising from a runner called a stolon
b. Single-tipped sporangiophores; no rhizoids or stolons; nonseptate hyphae, which show branching
c. Widespread in environment; conidia may be inhaled; microscopic appearance in specimen reveals dichotomous branching and septate hyphae
d. Yeast forms with budding blastoconidia often showing pseudohyphae; positive germ tube test; chlamydospores present

340. *Mucor* is best described by which of the following statements?

a. Round, black sporangia filled with endospores; sporangia unbranched, rising from a runner called a stolon
b. Single-tipped sporangiophores; no rhizoids or stolons; nonseptate hyphae, which show branching
c. Widespread in environment; conidia may be inhaled; microscopic appearance in specimen reveals dichotomous branching and septate hyphae
d. Yeast forms with budding blastoconidia often showing pseudohyphae; positive germ tube test; chlamydospores present

341. *Rhizopus* is best described by which of the following statements?

a. Round, black sporangia filled with endospores; sporangia unbranched, rising from a runner called a stolon
b. Single-tipped sporangiophores; no rhizoids or stolons; nonseptate hyphae, which show branching
c. Widespread in environment; conidia may be inhaled; microscopic appearance in specimen reveals dichotomous branching and septate hyphae
d. Yeast forms with budding blastoconidia often showing pseudohyphae; positive germ tube test; chlamydospores present

342. A 37-year-old Asian male was admitted to the hospital complaining of shortness of breath. He denied use of cigarettes, although did admit a previous history of intravenous drug abuse. His chest films showed a diffuse ground glass pattern. A specimen was obtained by bronchoalveolar lavage, and distinctive thin-walled trophozoites and thick-walled spherical cysts containing four to eight nucleii were observed using methenamine-silver stain. The most likely diagnosis of his illness is which of the following?

a. AIDS-related lymphoma
b. Aspergillosis
c. Blastomycosis
d. Histoplasmosis
e. *P. carinii* pneumonia

343. An 18-year-old white male high school student visited the school clinic complaining of a diffuse, painful rash extending from his midthigh to his navel region. He indicates that one of his football teammates gave him topical hydrocortisone to initially treat a minor groin rash. A KOH scraping of the lesion revealed the organisms shown in the accompanying picture. What is the most likely diagnosis of his rash?

Epidermophyton floccosum

(*Reproduced, with permission, from Brooks GF et al. Jawetz's Medical Microbiology, 22e. New York: McGraw-Hill, 2001, 536.*)

a. Coccidioidomycosis
b. Herpes simplex infection
c. Herpes zoster infection
d. Secondary syphilis
e. Tinea corporis (incognito)

344. A medical student was serving as a missionary in Africa. While assisting with the construction of a water project, a thorn pierced the glove of his left hand. Several days after the inflammation from the initial wound subsided, necrotizing lesions began to form that spread toward the elbow. Which of the following is the most likely etiological agent?

a. C. immitis
b. Malassezia furfur
c. M. canis
d. S. schenkii
e. Stachybotrys chartarum

Questions 345–349

345. Barrel-shaped arthroconidia are characteristics of which one of the following fungi?

a. Blastomyces dermatitidis
b. C. immitis
c. E. floccosum
d. M. canis
e. Phialophora verrucosa

346. Sporulation from flask-shaped, pigmented projections is commonly observed in which one of the following fungi?

a. B. dermatitidis
b. C. immitis
c. E. floccosum
d. M. canis
e. P. verrucosa

347. Clavate macroconidia are characteristic of which one of the following fungi?

a. B. dermatitidis
b. C. immitis
c. E. floccosum
d. M. canis
e. P. verrucosa

348. Broad-based budding cells are characteristic of which one of the following fungi?

a. *B. dermatitidis*
b. *C. immitis*
c. *E. floccosum*
d. *M. canis*
e. *P. verrucosa*

349. Rough-walled macroconidia of 8 to 15 cells are commonly observed in which one of the following fungi?

a. *B. dermatitidis*
b. *C. immitis*
c. *E. floccosum*
d. *M. canis*
e. *P. verrucosa*

Item 350–353

Fungal skin diseases may not be named according to the etiologic agent but rather are called *tinea* or a *dermatophytosis.*

350. Tinea corporis is caused by which of the following?

a. *E. floccosum*
b. *Exophiala werneckii*
c. *M. furfur*
d. *M. canis*
e. *Trichosporon beigelii*

351. Tinea pedis is caused by which of the following?

a. *E. floccosum*
b. *E. werneckii*
c. *M. furfur*
d. *M. canis*
e. *T. beigelii*

352. Tinea capitis is caused by which of the following?

a. *E. floccosum*
b. *E. werneckii*
c. *M. furfur*
d. *M. canis*
e. *T. beigelii*

353. Tinea versicolor is caused by which of the following?

a. *E. floccosum*
b. *E. werneckii*
c. *M. furfur*
d. *M. canis*
e. *T. beigelii*

354. A young man in his midtwenties presented with mucosal lesions in his mouth. Based on his CD4 cell count and other signs during the past few months, he was diagnosed as having AIDS. Which of the following is the most likely etiology of the oral lesions?

a. *Aspergillus*
b. *Candida*
c. *Cryptococcus*
d. *Mucor*
e. *Rhizopus*

Item 355–356

Harmless molds commonly seen growing on bread, as well as on a wide variety of other products or foodstuffs, grow equally well in the human host when the host's defenses are compromised.

355. It is difficult to determine whether isolation from one body site or body fluid is suggestive of colonization or infection. Which one of the following fungi is often isolated from blood, urine, and sputum in invasive disease?

a. *A. fumigatus*
b. *Basidiobolus ranarum*
c. *C. albicans*
d. *Conidiobolus coronata*
e. *Rhizopus arrhizus*

356. Which one of the following fungi causes rhinocerebral zygomycosis and is usually associated with acute diabetes?

a. *A. fumigatus*
b. *B. ranarum*
c. *C. albicans*
d. *C. coronata*
e. *R. arrhizus*

357. Three weeks after a patient with AIDS traveled to California to study desert flowers, he develops fever, chest pain, and muscle soreness. Two months later, red, tender nodules appear on the shins, and he has pain and tenderness in the right ankle. An x-ray film of the chest shows a left pleural effusion. What is the most likely diagnosis?

a. Blastomycosis
b. Coccidioidomycosis
c. Histoplasmosis
d. *Mycobacterium marinum* infection
e. *Mycoplasma pneumoniae* infection

358. Which of the following fungi is least likely to cause pulmonary disease?

a. *A. fumigatus*
b. *C. immitis*
c. *C. neoformans*
d. *H. capsulatum*
e. *S. schenckii*

359. An 18-year-old high school student in rural north Mississippi develops fever, cough, and chest pain. The cough, associated with weight loss, persisted. Because of poor performance at football practice, he was advised to see a physician. Lymph node biopsies stained with H and E studies revealed granulomatous inflammation and macrophages engorged with oval structures measuring 2 to 4 μ. Cultures incubated at room temperature grew powdery white colonies, which on microscopic study had tuberculate spores. The high school student acquired the infection from which of the following?

a. Another human via respiratory secretions
b. Bird excrement
c. Cat feces
d. Contaminated drinking water
e. Desert sand

Mycology

Answers

320. The answer is c. (*Brooks, pp 539–540, 551–553. Levinson, pp 304, 310–311. Murray—2002, pp 647, 661–662, 664–666. Ryan, pp 655–656, 660–664, 670–672.*) *C. neoformans* causes cryptococcosis, especially cryptococcal meningitis. The organisms can be seen in cerebrospinal fluid (CSF) in india ink preparations as an oval budding yeast surrounded by a wide, unstained polysaccharide capsule. *C. albicans,* the most important species of *Candida,* causes thrush and vaginitis, as well as other diseases. It may appear in tissue as a budding yeast or as elongated pseudohyphae (nonseptate). *S. schenckii* is a dimorphic fungus that appears as round or cigar-shaped budding yeasts in tissue. It causes a local pustule or ulcer that may become chronic.

321. The answer is a. (*Brooks, pp 553–554. Levinson, pp 312–313. Murray—2002, pp 667–668. Ryan, pp 665–667.*) *Aspergillus* species cause infections of the skin, eyes, and ears and "fungus ball" in the lungs. *Aspergillus* species occur only as molds (not dimorphic). They have septate hyphae that form V-shaped branches, whose walls are parallel. Septate, branching hyphae invading tissue are typically seen in biopsy. On culture, colonies with radiating chains of conidia (photo) are typical. These molds are widely spread in nature, and transmission is by airborne conidia. The organism is very opportunistic in immunocompromised individuals, and antifungal treatment may be difficult.

322. The answer is e. (*Brooks, pp 543, 545, 548. Levinson, pp 306–308. Murray—2002, p 652. Ryan, pp 674–678, 680–683.*) Thick-walled spores are characteristic of many fungal infections, including blastomycosis, coccidioidomycosis, and histoplasmosis. Observation of these structures in sputum or in tissue should alert the microbiologist to a diagnosis of systemic fungal infection. The presence of encapsulated yeast in clinical specimens may suggest the presence of *Cryptococcus*.

323. The answer is c. (*Brooks, p 537. Levinson, pp 303–304. Murray—2002, pp 642–646. Ryan, pp 649–650.*) Hairs infected with both M. canis and

M. audouini fluoresce with a yellow-green color under Wood's light, while *T. rubrum, T. tonsurans,* and *E. floccosum* do not. But *M. audouini* is an anthropophilic agent of tinea capitis, whereas *M. canis* is zoophilic. *M. canis* is seen primarily in children and is associated with infected cats or dogs.

324. The answer is b. (*Brooks, pp 552–553. Levinson, p 311. Murray—2002, pp 661–662. Ryan, pp 669–672.*) Patients with paralysis of their cellular immune system, such as in AIDS, are susceptible to a wide variety of diseases, including infection with *Cryptococcus.* A brain abscess caused by *C. neoformans* is not unusual in patients with AIDS. Initial laboratory suspicion is usually aroused by the presence of encapsulated yeast in the CSF. There also could be other microorganisms as well as noninfectious artifacts that superficially resemble yeast. While *C. neoformans* can be readily cultured, a rapid diagnosis can be made by detecting cryptococcal capsular polysaccharide in CSF or blood. Care must be taken to strictly control the test because rheumatoid factor may cross-react. Once the yeast is isolated, then specific stains as well as panels of assimilatory carbohydrates are available to definitively identify this organism as *C. neoformans.* The patient may also be infected with *P. carinii,* but not in the central nervous system. *P. carinii* has recently been reclassified as a fungus.

325. The answer is c. (*Brooks, pp 552–553. Levinson, p 311. Murray—2002, pp 661–662. Ryan, pp 669–672.*) *C. neoformans* occurs widely in nature, particularly in soil contaminated with bird droppings. Human infection occurs when inhalation of the organism occurs. Lung infection is often asymptomatic but can result in pneumonia. Meningitis occurs through dissemination, particularly in immunosuppressed patients. India ink preparations of CSF reveal a budding yeast with a wide, unstained capsule in infected persons.

326. The answer is e. (*Brooks, p 542. Levinson, p 304. Murray—2002, pp 648–649.*) Eumycotic mycetoma is a slowly progressing disease of the subcutaneous tissues that is caused by a variety of fungi. The term *Madura foot* has been used to describe the foot lesion. Although several fungi have been isolated in the United States from persons who have mycetoma, *Pseudallescheria boydii* appears to be one of the most common. Other foot infections that may resemble Madura foot are actinomycotic (bacterial) in nature. These are caused by *Nocardia brasiliensis* and *Actinomadura.*

327. The answer is d. (*Brooks, pp 543–549. Levinson, pp 305–308. Murray—2002, pp 651–656. Ryan, pp 672–683.*) Granuloma formation occurs in response to infection with many fungi. This cell-mediated immune response is seen in coccidioidomycosis, histoplasmosis, and blastomycosis, as well as in several others.

328. The answer is e. (*Brooks, pp 539–540. Levinson, p 304. Murray—2002, pp 647–648. Ryan, pp 654–656.*) Cutaneous sporotrichosis, caused by *S. schenckii*, begins at the site of inoculation, usually on an extremity or the face. The organism often is found on thorns of rosebushes. Ulceration is common, and new lesions appear along paths of lymphatic channels. Extracutaneous sporotrichosis is seen primarily in bones and joints. There is no evidence to suggest that any portal of entry besides skin is important.

329. The answer is b. (*Brooks, pp 535–538. Levinson, pp 303–304. Murray—2002, pp 642–646.*) The dermatophytes (see figure presented in the question) are a group of fungi that infect only superficial keratinized tissue (skin, hair, nails). They form hyphae and arthroconidia on the skin; in culture, they develop colonies and conidia. Tinea pedis, or athlete's foot, is the most common dermatophytosis. Several topical antifungal agents, such as undecylenic acid, salicylic acid, and ammoniated mercury, may be useful in treatment. For serious infection, systemic use of griseofulvin is effective.

330. The answer is e. (*Brooks, pp 550–552. Levinson, p 310. Murray—2002, pp 664–667. Ryan, pp 660–664.*) *C. albicans* is the most important species of *Candida* and causes thrush, vaginitis, skin and nail infections, and other infections. It is part of the normal flora of skin, mouth, GI tract, and vagina. It appears in tissues as an oval budding yeast or elongated pseudohyphae. It grows well on laboratory media and is identified by germ-tube formation. A vaccine is not available, and serologic and skin tests have little value.

331. The answer is b. (*Brooks, pp 550–552. Levinson, p 310. Murray—2002, pp 664–667. Ryan, pp 660–664.*) *C. albicans* is part of the normal flora of the gastrointestinal tract, mouth, and genital surfaces. Notwithstanding, *C. albicans* causes severe disease, particularly in those patients with compromised immunity. It is generally thought that when *C. albicans* is unable to adhere to mucosa it is nonpathogenic and that production of germ tubes or hyphae plays a major role in colonization and infection of the mucosal epithelial cells by allowing direct penetration of these cells with specific hydrolytic enzymes. While other mutations such as temperature intolerance, metabolic alterations, and structural substitutions may affect the ability of *Candida* to survive, these changes would not affect adherence.

332. The answer is a. (*Brooks, pp 553–554. Levinson, p 312. Murray— 2002, pp 607–609. Ryan, pp 665–667.*) While all fungi such as *Candida* and *Cryptococcus* are potentially serious in a bone marrow transplant unit (BMTU), the most frequent cause of fungal infection and death is *Aspergillus*. Aspergilli are ubiquitous in the environment. There are instances of multiple infections in new units that have not been monitored prior to opening or in units adjacent to construction projects. Strict precautions should be taken to exclude dust and debris from the BMTU area during construction, but in any event the environment should be monitored for airborne microorganisms, especially *Aspergillus,* prior to opening the unit.

333. The answer is b. (*Brooks, pp 545–547. Levinson, pp 306–307. Murray—2002, pp 651–655. Ryan, pp 672–676.*) *H. capsulatum* is a dimorphic fungus that forms two types of spores: tuberculate macroconidia and microconidia. Inhalation of the microconidia transmits infection. Inhaled spores (microconidia) are engulfed by macrophages and develop into yeast forms. Most infections remain asymptomatic; small granulomatous foci heal by calcification. However, pneumonia can occur. The heterophile antibody test is useful for early diagnosis of infectious mononucleosis.

334. The answer is d. (*Brooks, pp 542–544. Levinson, pp 305–306. Murray—2002, pp 659–661. Ryan, pp 678–680.*) *C. immitis* is a dimorphic fungus endemic in the southwestern United States. Arthrospores found in the soil are inhaled and infect the lungs, forming large, thick-walled spherules filled with endospores. A cell-mediated immune response results in asymptomatic infection in most people. Dissemination can occur in immunocompromised persons. A delayed hypersensitivity, manifest as red nodules (erythema nodosum) on extensor surfaces such as the shins, is an indicator of good prognosis. A rising titer of complement-fixing (CF) antibodies indicates dissemination; a decrease in titer correlates with a response to therapy.

335. The answer is c. *(Brooks, pp 543–545. Levinson, pp 305–306. Murray—2002, pp 659–660. Ryan, pp 678–680.) C. albicans* and *C. tropicalis* are opportunistic fungi, and as part of the normal flora are not transmitted by inhalation. *C. immitis* is a dimorphic fungus, and inhalation of the spores transmits the infection. *Sporothrix* is also a dimorphic fungus, but its portal of entry is cutaneous. *Trychophyton* is a dermatophyte and one of the causes of athlete's foot.

336. The answer is a. *(Brooks, pp 553–554. Levinson, p 312. Murray—2002, pp 667–669. Ryan, pp 665–667.) Aspergillus* is an opportunistic pathogen that can invade wounds, burns, abraded skin, the cornea, and the outer ear. However, in immunocompromised patients, infection of the wound site is not common. *Aspergillus* does not cause urinary tract infection. In immunocompromised persons, invasive disease occurs. Blood vessel invasion can result in thrombosis and infarction. In pulmonary cavities (due to tuberculosis), "fungus ball" formation can occur, which can be seen on x-ray. Infection of the bronchi can result in allergic bronchopulmonary aspergillosis, characterized by asthmatic symptoms. Thrush is caused by *C. albicans*. Rashes are not usually seen with *Aspergillus* infection.

337. The answer is b. *(Brooks, pp 543–545. Levinson, pp 305–306. Murray—2002, pp 659–660. Ryan, pp 680–683.)* In patients with coccidioidomycosis, a positive skin test to coccidioidin appears 2 to 21 days after the appearance of disease symptoms and may persist for 20 years without reexposure to the fungus. A decrease in intensity of the skin response often occurs in clinically healthy people who move away from endemic areas. A negative skin test frequently is associated with disseminated disease. Complement-fixing (CF) immunoglobulin G (IgG) antibodies, which may not appear at all in mild disease, rise to a high titer in disseminated disease, a poor prognostic sign. For this reason, a persistent or rising CF titer combined with clinical symptoms indicates present or imminent dissemination. Rarely is the CF titer negative. Most persons infected with *C. immitis* are immune to reinfection.

338–341. The answers are 338-d, 339-c, 340-b, 341-a. *(Brooks, pp 550–555. Levinson, pp 310–312. Murray—2002, pp 664–669. Ryan, pp 660–668.)* Fungi that cause opportunistic infections are diverse, and most of them are represented in this group of questions. Infection occurs primarily in the compromised host with underlying diseases such as lymphoma, leukemia, and diabetes. Unfortunately, most of the opportunistic fungi that cause infection are commonly seen in the laboratory as contaminants.

Candidiasis is the most frequent opportunistic infection. While *C. albicans* is most commonly isolated, other species such as *C. tropicalis* and *Torulopsis glabrata* are also seen. The yeasts may be identified biochemically, but *C. albicans* is distinctive in that it produces germ tubes and chlamydospores.

Aspergillosis, caused by a number of species of *Aspergillus,* is characterized in direct smear by septate hyphae, dichotomously branched. *Aspergillus flavus* and *A. fumigatus* are often seen as saprophytes in the laboratory but also account for the major species isolated from patients with aspergillosis. Differentiation of species, as with the zygomycetes, is dependent upon isolation of the fungus and precise morphological examination.

Zygomycosis, a term referring to infection by members of the class Zygomycetes, is caused primarily by *Rhizopus, Mucor,* and *Absidia.* Other zygomycetes such as *Basidiobolus* and *Cunninghamella* are rarely encountered. The lack of septate hyphae on a direct smear may be the initial hint of zygomycosis. However, not uncommonly, the occasional hypha of *Mucor* will have a septa. The genera cannot be differentiated on a direct patient specimen. The organism must be isolated and slide cultures performed to observe the characteristic morphology of these filamentous fungi.

Rhizopus species have sporangia that arise from a stolon, while *Mucor* species do not. *Mucor* species have collarettes; *Rhizopus* species do not.

342. The answer is e. *(Brooks, p 555. Levinson, pp 324–325. Murray— 2002, pp 669–671. Ryan, pp 685–689.)* *P. carinii* causes pneumonia in immunocompromised patients. Once considered a protozoan, it is not classified as a fungus. Effective chemoprophylactic regimens have resulted in a dramatic decrease in pneumonia deaths in AIDS patients. *P. carinii* has the morphologically distinct forms (trophozoite and cyst) described in the question. Cysts stain well with silver stain. In clinical specimens, trophozoites and cysts are present in a tight mass. *P. carinii* cannot be cultured. The organism is widespread in nature and does not cause disease without immunosuppression. It may represent a member of normal flora.

343. The answer is e. *(Brooks, pp 535–538. Levinson, p 303. Murray—2002, pp 643–646. Ryan, p 653.)* Of the available answer choices, only tinea corporis dermatophyte infection will show numerous, smooth-walled macroconidia, with microconidia being absent. *Epidermophyton* species would be a common cause of this kind of rash. Jock itch (tinia cruruis—groin) can involve particularly bad lesions if inappropriate use of topical steroids is involved. This is also called tinea incognito. Tinea or ringworm designations were used because of the dermatophyte infections. Treatment usually consists of thorough removal of infected and dead epithelial structure and application of a topical antifungal medication.

344. The answer is d. *(Brooks, pp 531, 539–540. Levinson, p 304. Murray— 2002, pp 639–640. Ryan, pp 654–656.)* *S. schenkii* is a dimorphic fungus that lives on vegetation. A mold with branching septate hyphae and conidia at ambient temperature, it grows as a small budding yeast at 37°C. Following traumatic introduction into the skin, a chronic granulomatous infection occurs with secondary spread to local lymph nodes. For systemic treatment, Amphoteracin B is given. *Malassezia* and *Microsporum* produce superficial infections. *Coccidioides* would be transmitted by airborne mechanisms. *S. chartarum* is the toxic house mold that is so prevalent in current news reports.

345–349. The answers are 345-b, 346-e, 347-c, 348-a, 349-d. *(Brooks, pp 537, 540, 543, 548–549. Levinson, pp 303–307, 308. Murray— 2002, pp 640, 643–645, 655–656, 659–660. Ryan, pp 649–650, 676–683.)* Microscopic examination of fungal isolates is essential to the identification of the organism.

C. *immitis* is a dimorphic fungus endemic in some regions of the southwestern United States and in Latin America. In tissue, the organism exists as a spherule filled with endospores. When grown on solid media, the organism produces barrel-shaped arthroconidia, which stain with lactophenol cotton blue.

P. *verrucosa* is one of the causes of chromoblastomycosis, a chronic localized infection of the skin and subcutaneous tissue. Microscopically, short or somewhat elongated, flask-shaped, pigmented phialides are seen. The collarettes are vase-shaped and darkly pigmented.

Macroscopically, the colonies of *Epidermophyton* have a yellowish appearance. This fungus invades skin and nails but never hair. On microscopic examination, clavate or paddle-shaped macroconidia are evident, with rounded ends and smooth walls. Microconidia are absent.

B. *dermatitidis* causes a chronic granulomatous disease. The yeast cells are globose or ovoid in shape. The single blastoconidium is attached by broad base to the parent cell.

M. *canis* is a dermatophyte that infects skin and hair but rarely nails. When hair is infected with this organism, it will fluoresce. Microscopic examination of this organism demonstrates rough-walled macroconidia of 8 to 15 cells.

350–353. The answers are 350-d, 351-a, 352-d, 353-c. (*Brooks, pp 534–538. Levinson, pp 303–304. Murray—2002, pp 639–646. Ryan, pp 649–650, 654.*) Dermatomycoses are cutaneous mycoses caused by three genera of fungi: *Microsporum, Trichophyton,* and *Epidermophyton.* These infections are called *tinea* or *ringworm,* a misnomer that has persisted from the days when they were thought to be caused by worms or lice. Tinea capitis (ringworm of the scalp) is due to an infection with M. *canis* or T. *tonsurans.* It usually occurs during childhood and heals spontaneously at puberty. Circular areas on the scalp, with broken or no hair, are characteristic of this disorder. Tinea corporis (ringworm of the body) is caused by M. *canis* and *Trichophyton mentagrophytes.* This disorder affects smooth skin and produces circular pruritic areas of redness and scaling. Both tinea cruris (ringworm of the groin, "jock itch") and tinea pedis (ringworm of the feet, athlete's foot) are caused by T. *rubrum,* T. *mentagrophytes,* or E. *floccosum.* These common conditions are pruritic and can cause scaling. Tinea versicolor (pityriasis versicolor) is not a dermatomycotic condition but, rather, a superficial mycosis now thought to be caused by M. *furfur.* The disorder is characterized by chronic but asymptomatic scaling on the trunk, arms, or other parts of the body.

354. The answer is b. (*Brooks, pp 550–554. Levinson, pp 310–312. Murray—2002, pp 661–668. Ryan, pp 660–664.*) *Candida* species are normal flora of the skin, mucous membranes, and gastrointestinal tract. The risk of endogenans infection is ever present. Candidiasis is the most common systemic mycosis. Oral thrush develops in most patients with AIDS. Other risk factors include antibiotic use and cellular immunodeficiency. *Mucor* and *Rhizopus* are primarily dermatophytes, while *Aspergillus* is usually derived from an environmental source. While *Aspergillus* is a significant opportunist, the numbers of cases are much lower than those observed to be caused by *Candida. Cryptococcus* is usually acquired by inhalation.

355–356.   The answers are 355-c, 356-e. *(Brooks, pp 550–556. Levinson, pp 310–312. Murray—2002, pp 664–672.)* Candidiasis, cryptococcosis, zygomycosis, and aspergillosis are among the most common opportunistic fungal infections. These fungi are commonly observed in the environment and are innocuous to people with intact host defenses. However, when host defenses are compromised by immunosuppression (AIDS), cytotoxic drugs, diabetes, or devices that breach the normal host defenses, these usually harmless fungi become potent pathogenic microorganisms.

C. albicans is a member of the normal human microflora. This yeast causes such relatively mild infections as "jock itch" and diaper rash. Suppression of cellular immunity often results in more serious yeast infections. Oral candidiasis is one of the earliest and most frequent of the opportunistic infections in patients with AIDS. Diagnosis of invasive candidiasis is difficult, especially when patients are symptomatic and *Candida* is not recovered from blood specimens. Candidal antibody tests, antigen detection, and metabolite detection have not been successful in differentiating between invasive disease and colonization. The figure presented in question 338 illustrates *C. albicans* from a skin smear. Zygomycosis (sometimes called *mucormycosis*) is caused by a variety of fungi called zygomycetes. These fungi include *Conidiobolus, Rhizopus,* and *Basidiobolus,* which can be differentiated mycologically, but all are characterized by large (6 to 25 mm), irregularly branched, usually nonseptate hyphae. The differentiation of these fungi clinically is a function of the location of the lesion: limbs and trunk, nose, or brain. *Basidiobolus* lesions are most commonly seen on the arms and legs. *Conidiobolus* is usually found in the nasal mucosa and nasal sinuses. *Rhizopus* infection may start in the nasal tissue but spreads rapidly to the eyes and brain.

357.   The answer is b. *(Brooks, pp 543–545. Levinson, pp 305–306. Murray—2002, pp 659–660. Ryan, pp 678–683.)* Endemic areas for *C. immitis* are semi-arid regions, particularly the central valleys of California and southern Arizona. The infection rate is highest during the dry months of summer and autumn, when dust is prevalent. Inhalation of arthroconidia can lead to an asymptomatic infection in 60% of individuals. The other 40% may develop a self-limited influenza-like illness. Individuals with cell-mediated immunosuppression may lead to dissemination of endospores by the blood. The most frequent sites involved are skin, bones and joints, and the meninges. Histoplasmosis is usually associated with the central river valleys of the United

States, while blastomycocis is endemic primarily in the eastern United States. *M. marinum* is usually associated with fish and water, while *M. pneumoniae* transmission is from person to person.

358. The answer is e. *(Brooks, pp 539–540. Levinson, p 304. Murray— 2002, p 647. Ryan, pp 654–656.) Sporothrix* is a dimorphic fungus that lives on vegetation. While a mold form at ambient temperatures and producing septate hyphae and conidia, the infection almost always follows traumatic introduction into the skin. A chronic granulomatus infection is typical, with local lymph nodes being involved. Multiple lesions (abscesses) may occur along the lymphatics. *Histoplasma, Coccidioides, Cryptococcus,* and *Aspergillus* are usually acquired by inhalation.

359. The answer is b. *(Brooks, pp 545–548. Levinson, pp 306–307. Murray— 2002, pp 651–654. Ryan, pp 672–676.) H. capsulatum* infection is highest in the United States, especially in the Ohio and Mississippi river valleys. Numerous outbreaks have resulted from exposure of many persons to inocula of conidia. These occur when the organism is disturbed from its natural habitat, soil mixed with bird feces or bat guano. Feces provides an excellent culture for fungal growth to occur. Some 80 to 90% of residents in certain endemic areas may have positive skin tests. Histoplasmosis is not transmissible from person to person.

Parasitology

Questions

DIRECTIONS: Each question below contains four or more suggested responses. Select the **one best** response to each question.

360. Babesiosis, as observed in the figure below, is a tick-borne disease resulting in a febrile illness. Infection with *Babesia* is most commonly observed in which of the following?

(*Photomicrograph by Zane Price. Reproduced, with permission, from Markell EK, Voge M, and John DT:* Medical Parasitology, *6e. Philadelphia: W.B. Saunders Co., 1986.*)

a. AIDS patients
b. Foresters
c. Patients without a spleen
d. Transfusion recipients
e. Transplant recipients

361. An AIDS patient presents to his primary care physician with a two-week history of watery, nonbloody diarrhea. This stool revealed an organism that can be seen in the figure below. The most likely diagnosis is which of the following?

(*Reproduced, with permission, from Garcia LS:* Laboratory Methods for Diagnosis of Parasitic Infection. *In Baron EJ and Finegold SM:* Diagnostic Microbiology, *8e. St. Louis: Mosby-Year Book, 1990.*)

a. Acid-fast bacilli
b. *Enterocytozoon*
c. *Cryptosporidium*
d. *Cyclospora*
e. Yeast

362. A person who had recently consumed half a box of raspberries came down with severe watery diarrhea. Surprisingly, the patient felt tired for a few days and had a low-grade fever. What is the most likely cause of infection?

a. *Escherichia coli* 0157:H7
b. *Cyclospora*
c. *Cryptosporidium*
d. *Isospora*
e. *Vibrio*

363. In order to exert control over the primary cause of toxoplasmosis of pregnancy, which one of the following steps of the life cycle of *Toxoplasma* would be most practical to interrupt?

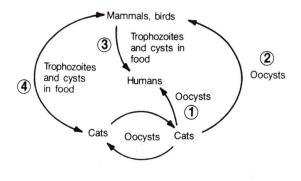

a. Step 1
b. Step 2
c. Step 3
d. Step 4
e. Steps 3 and 4

364. A 30-year-old female stored her contact lenses in tap water. She noticed deterioration of vision and visited an ophthalmologist, who diagnosed her with severe retinitis. Culture of the water as well as vitreous fluid would most likely reveal which one of the following?

a. *Acanthamoeba*
b. *Babesia*
c. *Entamoeba coli*
d. *Naegleria*
e. *Pneumocystis*

365. The diagnostic characteristics of *Plasmodium falciparum* (see figure) are best described by which one of the following statements?

(*Reproduced, with permission, from Garcia LS:* Laboratory Methods for Diagnosis of Parasitic Infection. *In Baron EJ and Finegold SM:* Diagnostic Microbiology, *8e. St. Louis: Mosby-Year Book, 1990.*)

a. An important diagnostic feature is the irregular appearance of the edges of the infected red blood cell
b. A period of 72 hours is required for the development of the mature schizont, which resembles a rosette with only 8 to 10 oval merozoites
c. Except in infections with very high parasitemia, only ring forms of early trophozoites and the gametocytes are seen in the peripheral blood
d. Schüffner stippling is routinely seen in red blood cells that harbor parasites
e. The signet-ring-shaped trophozoite is irregular in shape with ameboid extensions of the cytoplasm

366. The life cycle of this parasite consists of two stages: the cyst and the trophozoite, as shown in the figure below. What is the most likely identification of this organism?

(Reproduced, with permission, from Garcia LS: Laboratory Methods for Diagnosis of Parasitic Infections. *In Baron EJ and Finegold SM:* Diagnostic Microbiology, *8e. St. Louis: Mosby-Year Book, 1990.)*

a. *Clonorchis*
b. *Entamoeba*
c. *Giardia*
d. *Pneumocystis*
e. *Trichomonas*

367. A divorced working mother takes her 4-year-old child to a day-care center. She has noticed that the child's frequent stools are nonbloody with mucus and are foul smelling. The child has no fever, but does complain of "tummy hurting." The increase of fat in the stool directs the pediatrician's concern toward a diagnosis of malabsorption syndrome associated with which of the following?

a. Amebiasis
b. Ascariasis
c. Balantidiasis
d. Enterobiasis
e. Giardiasis

368. Human infection with the beef tapeworm, *Taenia saginata,* usually is less serious than infection with the pork tapeworm, *Taenia solium,* because of which of the following statements?

a. Acute intestinal stoppage is less common in beef tapeworm infection
b. Beef tapeworm eggs cause less irritation of the mucosa of the digestive tract
c. Larval invasion does not occur in beef tapeworm infection
d. The adult beef tapeworms are smaller
e. Toxic by-products are not given off by the adult beef tapeworm

369. A man coughed up a long (4 to 6 cm) white worm, and his chief complaint was abdominal tenderness. He reports that he goes to sushi bars at least once a week. The following parasites have been observed in people who eat raw fish: *Anisakis, Pseudoterranova, Eustrongylides,* and *Angiostrongylus.* Which of the following would best differentiate the specific parasitic agent?

a. Antigen detection in tissues
b. Characteristic signs and symptoms
c. Identification of specific species of fish involved
d. Specific antibody tests
e. Study of distinctive morphology of the parasite

370. A survey of 100 healthy adults reveals that 80% have IgG antibodies to *Toxoplasma*. Which one of the following statements would help to explain this finding?

a. A variety of parasitic infections induce the formation of *Toxoplasma* antibody
b. The IgM test is more reliable than the IgG test for determination of past infections; retesting for IgM would show that most people do not have *Toxoplasma* antibody
c. The potential for *Toxoplasma* infection is widespread, and the disease is mild and self-limiting
d. The test for *Toxoplasma* antibodies is highly nonspecific
e. Toxoplasmosis is caused by eating meat; therefore, all meat eaters have had toxoplasmosis

371. In the United States, certain enteric protozoan and helminthic infections were previously considered to be exotic illnesses related to foreign travel or to contaminated food or water. However, sexual transmission of these diseases has produced a "hyperendemic" infection rate among male homosexuals. The most common infection seen in this group is which of the following?

a. Amebiasis
b. Ascariasis
c. Enterobiasis
d. Giardiasis
e. Trichuriasis

372. Analysis of a patient's stool reveals small structures resembling rice grains; microscopic examination shows these to be proglottids. What is the most likely organism in this patient's stool?

a. *Ascaris lumbricoides*
b. *Enterobius vermicularis*
c. *Necator americanus*
d. *T. saginata*
e. *Trichuris trichiura*

373. An AIDS patient complains of headaches and disorientation. A clinical diagnosis of *Toxoplasma encephalitis* is made and *Toxoplasma* cysts were observed in a brain section (see figure below). Which one of the following antibody results would be most likely in this patient?

a. IgM nonreactive, IgG nonreactive
b. IgM nonreactive, IgG reactive (low titer)
c. IgM reactive (low titer), IgG reactive (high titer)
d. IgM reactive (high titer), IgG reactive (high titer)
e. IgM reactive (high titer), IgG nonreactive

374. *Trypanosoma cruzi* initially penetrates through the mucous membranes on the skin and then multiplies in a lesion known as a *chagoma*. In the chronic stage of the disease, where are the main lesions often observed?

a. Digestive tract and respiratory tract
b. Heart and digestive tract
c. Heart and liver
d. Liver and spleen
e. Spleen and pancreas

375. A woman, recently returned from Africa, complains of having paroxysmal attacks of chills, fever, and sweating. These attacks last a day or two at a time and recur every 36 to 48 hours. Examination of a stained blood specimen reveals ringlike and crescent-like forms within red blood cells. Which of the following is the most likely infecting organism?

a. *Plasmodium falciparum*
b. *Plasmodium vivax*
c. *Schistosoma mansoni*
d. *Trypanosoma gambiense*
e. *Wuchereria bancrofti*

Item 376–377

A young man, recently returned to the United States from Vietnam, has severe liver disease. Symptoms include jaundice, anemia, and weakness.

376. Which of the following is the etiologic agent, shown in the photomicrographs below?

a. *Clonorchis sinensis*
b. *Diphyllobothrium latum*
c. *P. falciparum*
d. *T. saginata*
e. *T. solium*

377. An intermediate form of the organism shown in the above photomicrographs lives in which of the following organisms?

a. Cows
b. Mosquitoes
c. Pigs
d. Snails
e. Ticks

378. A woman who recently traveled through Central Africa now complains of severe chills and fever, abdominal tenderness, and darkening urine. Her febrile periods last for 28 hours and recur regularly. Which of the blood smears drawn below would most likely be associated with the symptoms described?

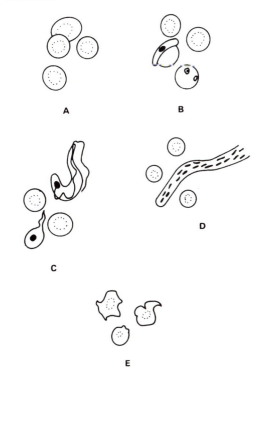

A

B

C

D

E

a. A
b. B
c. C
d. D
e. E

379. One of the most clinically significant infections in patients with AIDS is *Pneumocystis carinii* pneumonia (PCP). PCP is a treatable disease; therefore, rapid diagnosis is essential. The method of choice for detection of *P. carinii* in respiratory specimens is which of the following?

a. Culture in rat lung cells
b. Direct fluorescent antibody (DFA) microscopy
c. Indirect fluorescent antibody (IFA) microscopy
d. Methenamine-silver stain
e. Toluidine blue stain

380. Which of the following protozoa is known only in the trophozoite stage?

a. *Balantidium coli*
b. *Entamoeba histolytica*
c. *Giardia lamblia*
d. *Taxoplasma gondii*
e. *Trichomonas vaginalis*

381. An international photographer returns to the United States from a global picture assignment. He is seen by his physician, giving his major complaint as diarrhea. Which of the following can be ruled out?

a. *Echinococcus granulosus*
b. *Dientamoeba fragilis*
c. *D. latum*
d. *G. lamblia*
e. *Leishmania donovani*

382. A "parasite" that may be a fungus is the initial clinical manifestation in up to 60% of patients with AIDS. What is this organism?

a. Blastocystis
b. *Blastomyces*
c. *Cryptosporidium*
d. Microsporidium
e. *Pneumocystis*

383. A medical technologist visited Scandinavia and consumed raw fish daily for two weeks. Six months after her return home, she had a routine physical and was found to be anemic. Her vitamin B_{12} levels were below normal. What is the most likely cause of her vitamin B_{12} deficiency anemia?

a. Cysticercosis
b. Excessive consumption of ice-cold vodka
c. Infection with the fish tapeworm *D. latum*
d. Infection with Parvovirus B19
e. Infection with *Yersinia*

384. A renal transplant patient was admitted for graft rejection and pneumonia. A routine evaluation of his stool showed rhabditiform larvae. Subsequent follow-up revealed similar worms in his sputum. He had no eosinophils in his peripheral circulation. What is the most likely organism?

a. *Ascaris*
b. *Hymenolepis*
c. *Loa loa*
d. *Necator*
e. *Strongyloides*

385. Which of the following best describes lice?

a. *Pediculus humanus* is the only species of louse
b. They cause tissue edema
c. They have wings
d. They secrete a potent neurotoxin
e. They transmit epidemic typhus, relapsing fever, and trench fever

386. Malaria is a significant worldwide public health problem. The life cycle of *Plasmodium* can be seen in the figure below. Which one of the following control methods for malaria is currently effective?

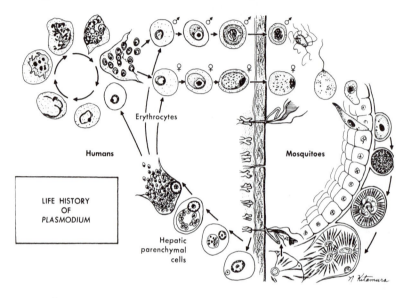

a. Antibiotics
b. A vaccine
c. Chemoprophylaxis
d. Tick repellents
e. White clothing

387. Scabies is caused by a small mite that burrows into the skin. The disease is best described by which one of the following statements?

a. Allergic (asthma-like) reactions to mites are rare
b. It is best diagnosed by biopsy of the inflammatory region around the mite bite
c. It is caused by a species of *Sarcoptes*
d. It is synonymous with Kawasaki's syndrome
e. Secondary bacterial infection is rare

388. Amebas that are parasitic in humans are found in the oral cavity and the intestinal tract. Which one of the following statements best describes these intestinal amebas?

a. Infection with *E. histolytica* is limited to the intestinal tract
b. They are usually nonpathogenic
c. They are usually transmitted as trophozoites
d. They can cause peritonitis and liver abscesses
e. They occur most abundantly in the duodenum

389. Schistosomiasis is a disease characterized by granulomatous reactions to the ova or to products of the parasite at the place of oviposition. Clinical manifestations include which one of the following?

a. Arthropathies
b. Bladder wall hyperplasia
c. Cardiac abnormalities
d. Pulmonary embolism
e. Splenomegaly

390. *Borrelia burgdorferi*, the causative agent of Lyme disease, has been isolated from a variety of ticks such as *Ixodes scapularis, Amblyomma, Dermacentor,* and *Ixodes pacificus*. Which one of the following statements is true of Lyme disease?

a. *Dermacentor* and *Amblyomma* are significant vectors of *B. burgdorferi* to humans
b. Dogs and cats are naturally immune to Lyme disease
c. *I. scapularis* and *Ixodes dammini* are different types of ticks
d. Only a small percentage of people who get bitten by a tick develop Lyme disease
e. White-tailed deer, an important reservoir for *I. scapularis,* are dying because of Lyme disease

391. Which of the following infections requires a mosquito for transmission to humans?

a. Babesiosis
b. Bancroftian filariasis
c. Dog tapeworm
d. Guinea worm
e. Leishmaniasis

Item 392–395

Flukes (trematodes) have a great impact on worldwide public health, causing both morbidity and mortality.

392. Which of the following organisms penetrates skin, is endemic in Africa and Latin America, and has a large lateral spine on its eggs?

a. *Clonorchis*
b. *Paragonimus*
c. *Schistosoma haematobium*
d. *Schistosoma japonicum*
e. *S. mansoni*

393. Which of the following organisms may be ingested with raw fish, affects the liver, and has an operculated egg?

a. *Clonorchis*
b. *Paragonimus*
c. *S. haematobium*
d. *S. japonicum*
e. *S. mansoni*

394. Which of the following organisms penetrates skin, is endemic in Asia, and has a small lateral spine on its eggs?

a. *Clonorchis*
b. *Paragonimus*
c. *S. haematobium*
d. *S. japonicum*
e. *S. mansoni*

395. Which of the following organisms penetrates skin, is endemic in Africa and the Middle East, has large terminal spines on its eggs, and is found in urine samples?

a. *Clonorchis*
b. *Paragonimus*
c. *S. haematobium*
d. *S. japonicum*
e. *S. mansoni*

Item 396–399

A primary procedure for diagnosis of fecal parasites is a stained smear of feces. For some parasitic infections, however, other specimens may be more productive.

396. *G. lamblia* is best diagnosed by which of the following?

a. Baermann technique
b. Dilution followed by egg count
c. Enzyme immunoassay (EIA)
d. Examination of a cellophane tape swab
e. Sigmoidoscopy and aspiration of mucosal lesions

397. *E. histolytica* infection is best diagnosed by which of the following?

a. Baermann technique
b. Dilution followed by egg count
c. Enzyme immunoassay (EIA)
d. Examination of a cellophane tape swab
e. Sigmoidoscopy and aspiration of mucosal lesions

398. The best method for the detection of *Strongyloides* larvae is which of the following?

a. Baermann technique
b. Dilution followed by egg count
c. Enzyme immunoassay (EIA)
d. Examination of a cellophane tape swab
e. Sigmoidoscopy and aspiration of mucosal lesions

399. *Ascaris* is best observed in human specimens by which one of the following?

a. Baermann technique
b. Dilution followed by egg count
c. Enzyme immunoassay (EIA)
d. Examination of a cellophane tape swab
e. Sigmoidoscopy and aspiration of mucosal lesions

Questions 400–403

400. A butcher who is fond of eating raw hamburger develops chorioretinitis; a Sabin-Feldman dye test is positive. This patient is most likely infected with which of the following?

a. Giardiasis
b. Schistosomiasis
c. Toxoplasmosis
d. Trichinosis
e. Visceral larva migrans

401. A fur trapper complains of sore muscles, has swollen eyes, and reports eating bear meat on a regular basis. He is at risk for which one of the following?

a. Giardiasis
b. Schistosomiasis
c. Toxoplasmosis
d. Trichinosis
e. Visceral larva migrans

402. A newspaper correspondent has diarrhea for two weeks following a trip to St. Petersburg (Leningrad). You might expect her to have which one of the following?

a. Giardiasis
b. Schistosomiasis
c. Toxoplasmosis
d. Trichinosis
e. Visceral larva migrans

403. A retired Air Force colonel has had abdominal pain for two years; he makes yearly freshwater fishing trips to Puerto Rico and often wades with bare feet into streams. Which of the following should be in your differential diagnosis?

a. Giardiasis
b. Schistosomiasis
c. Toxoplasmosis
d. Trichinosis
e. Visceral larva migrans

404. A teenager who works in a dog kennel after school has had a skin rash, eosinophilia, and an enlarged liver and spleen for two years. What is the most likely cause of this infection?

a. Giardiasis
b. Schistosomiasis
c. Toxoplasmosis
d. Trichinosis
e. Visceral larva migrans

Item 405–409

Certain parasites are found most commonly in particular body contents.

405. A protozoan with characteristic jerky motility is most commonly observed in which of the following?

a Biopsied muscle
b. Blood
c. Duodenal contents
d. Sputum
e. Vaginal secretions

406. A helminth that is naturally transmitted by ingestion of pork, bear, or walrus meat could be detected in which of the following?

a. Biopsied muscle
b. Blood
c. Duodenal contents
d. Sputum
e. Vaginal secretions

407. A tissue-dwelling trematode that may be found in feces can also be detected in which of the following?

a. Biopsied muscle
b. Blood
c. Duodenal contents
d. Sputum
e. Vaginal secretions

408. Cysts of a protozoan adhere to a piece of nylon yarn coiled in a gelatin capsule, which is swallowed. These cysts are usually found in which of the following?

a. Biopsied muscle
b. Blood
c. Duodenal contents
d. Sputum
e. Vaginal secretions

409. A parasite resembling malaria that infects both animals and humans and is carried by the same tick that transmits B. *burgdorferi* (the bacterium that causes Lyme disease) would most likely be observed in which of the following?

a. Biopsied muscle
b. Blood
c. Duodenal contents
d. Sputum
e. Vaginal secretions

Parasitology

Answers

360. The answer is c. *(Brooks, p 580. Levinson, p 330. Murray—2002, pp 716–717.)* *Babesia* is a tick-borne organism transmitted by *I. scapularis*, the same tick that transmits Lyme disease. *Babesia* is often mistaken for *Plasmodia* (causative organism of malaria) on a blood smear. Patients become anemic and develop hepatosplenomegaly, but patients who are asplenic are at a much greater risk. Transfusion recipients, foresters, and immunosuppressed patients may be at risk of acquiring disease but not to the same extent as those patients who have been splenectomized.

361. The answer is c. *(Brooks, p 582. Levinson, p 319. Murray—2002, pp 706–707. Ryan, p 702.)* The figure presented in the question shows a *Cryptosporidium* oocyst stained with a fluorescent-labeled specific antibody. *Cryptosporidium* may also be stained with a modified acid-fast stain but are not acid-fast bacilli. They are smaller than *Cyclospora*, which are yeast size, but larger than *Enterocytozoon*, one of the microsporidia.

362. The answer is b. *(Levinson, pp 330–331. Murray—2002, pp 707–709.)* Cyclosporiasis is a newly recognized food- and water-borne infectious disease associated with eating contaminated berries imported from some Central American countries. *Cyclospora* are moderately acid-fast but twice the size of *Cryptosporidium*. Patients usually have frequent diarrhea for up to three weeks and usually suffer only malaise and fatigue. The disease is self-limiting, but relapses can occur.

363. The answer is a. *(Brooks, pp 582–584. Levinson, pp 323–324. Murray—2002, pp 717–720. Ryan, pp 722–727.)* *T. gondii* may be acquired by inhalation of oocysts in cat feces. It is difficult to control the habits of cats unless they are housed and not let out. Pregnant human females should avoid changing cat litter boxes. While ingestion of oocysts in raw meat may also lead to toxoplasmosis, inhalation of oocysts is the primary cause, particularly among pregnant women in the United States.

364. The answer is a. *(Brooks, p 575. Levinson, p 330. Murray—2002, pp 720–721. Ryan, p 733.)* Acanthamoeba is a free-living ameba, as is Naegleria. Naegleria usually causes severe, often fatal, meningoencephalitis, while Acanthamoeba is uncommonly isolated from contact lens fluid and patients with retinitis who do not store their lenses under sterile conditions. Acanthamoeba can be grown on nonnutrient agar plates using E. coli as a food source. They are identified microscopically with use of a nonspecific fluorescent stain.

365. The answer is c. *(Brooks, pp 575–580. Levinson, pp 321–323. Murray—2002, pp 715–716. Ryan, p 712.)* P. falciparum infection is distinguished by the appearance of ring forms of early trophozoites and gametocytes, both of which can be found in the peripheral blood. The size of the RBC is usually normal. Double dots in the rings are common.

366. The answer is c. *(Brooks, pp 562–563. Levinson, pp 318–319. Murray—2002, pp 701–703. Ryan, pp 745–748.)* Giardia exists in both trophozoite and cyst form. The "trophs" are fragile and not commonly seen in stools. The cysts are infectious. Giardia is the most common parasitic disease in the United States. It is commonly contracted from drinking cyst-contaminated water. Chlorine does not kill Giardia cysts, but contaminated water can be made cyst-free by filtration.

367. The answer is e. *(Brooks, pp 562–563. Levinson, pp 318–319. Murray—2002, pp 701–703. Ryan, pp 745–748.)* G. lamblia is the only common protozoan found in the duodenum and jejenum. Tropozoites are commonly found in the duodenum and do not penetrate the tissues. Four nucleii cysts (infective stage) can remain viable for up to four months. Excystation is via digestive enzymes. The mechanical irritation to tissues leads to diarrhea, with increased fat and mucus in the foul-smelling stool. Malabsorption syndrome (vitamin A and fats) leads to weight loss, anorexia, electrolyte imbalance, and abdominal cramps. Children and immunocompromised individuals are most significantly affected. Giardiasis should be considered in the differential diagnosis of any "traveler's diarrhea."

368. The answer is c. *(Brooks, pp 593–594. Levinson, pp 332–335. Murray—2002, pp 754–757. Ryan, pp 793–797.)* Both beef tapeworm (T. sagi-

nata) and pork tapeworm (*T. solium*) can, in the adult form, cause disturbances of intestinal function. Intestinal disorder is due not only to direct irritation but also to the action of metabolic toxic wastes. In addition, *T. saginata*, because of its large size, may produce acute intestinal blockage. Unlike *T. saginata*, *T. solium* produces cysticercosis, which results in serious lesions in humans (in *T. saginata*, the cysticercus—encysted larvae stage—develops only in cattle).

369. The answer is e. (*Brooks, p 586. Levinson, p 352.*) The consumption of raw fish products in Asian restaurants, especially the growing popularity of sushi and sashimi, has led to a variety of infections, most of which are characterized by symptoms consistent with intestinal blockage or meningitis. The parasites are tissue nematodes and parasites of marine mammals. Fish, squid, and other edible marine life are often secondary hosts. The most reliable way to differentiate the specific helminth is by examination of the whole worm or by histologic examination of the parasites in tissue sections.

370. The answer is c. (*Brooks, pp 582–584. Levinson, pp 323–324. Murray—2002, pp 717–720. Ryan, pp 722–727.*) Serologic tests, such as the Sabin-Feldman dye test and indirect immunofluorescence, have shown that a high percentage of the world's population has been infected with *T. gondii*. In adults, clinical toxoplasmosis usually presents as a benign syndrome resembling infectious mononucleosis. However, fetal infections are often severe and associated with hydrocephalus, chorioretinitis, convulsions, and death. Acute toxoplasmosis is best diagnosed by an IgM capture assay. In most patients, specific IgM antibody disappears within three to six months.

371. The answer is d. (*Brooks, pp 562–563. Levinson, pp 318–319. Murray—2002, pp 701–703. Ryan, pp 745–748.*) The infection rate with *G. lamblia* in male homosexuals has been reported to be from 21 to 40%. These high prevalence rates are probably related to three factors: the endemic rate, the sexual behavior that facilitates transmission (the usual barriers to spread have been interrupted), and the frequency of exposure to an infected person.

372. The answer is d. (*Brooks, pp 593–594. Levinson, pp 332–335. Murray—2002, pp 754–757. Ryan, pp 793–795.*) *Enterobius* (pinworm), *Ascaris* (roundworm), *Necator* (hookworm), and *Trichuris* (whipworm) are roundworms, or nematodes. *T. saginata* (tapeworm), a segmented flatworm, affects the small intestine of humans. Tapeworm segments, called *proglottids*, appear in the stool of infected persons.

373. The answer is b. (*Brooks, pp 582–584. Levinson, pp 323–324. Murray—2002, pp 717–720. Ryan, pp 722–727.*) One of the leading causes of death among AIDS patients is central nervous system toxoplasmosis. It is thought that *Toxoplasma* infection is a result of reactivation of old or preexisting toxoplasmosis. Occasionally, the infection may be acquired by needle sharing. Because the disease is a reactivation of old or preexisting toxoplasmosis, routine quantitative tests for IgM antibody are usually negative and IgG titers are low (≤1:256, IFA). More sophisticated methods, such as IgM capture or IgG avidity, may reveal an acute response.

374. The answer is b. (*Brooks, pp 565, 568–570. Levinson, pp 325–326. Murray—2002, pp 725–727. Ryan, pp 695, 757–760.*) American trypanosomiasis (Chagas' disease) is produced by *T. cruzi*, which is transmitted to humans by the bite of an infected reduviid bug. After multiplication, the tissues most likely to be affected in the chronic stage of the disease are the cardiac muscle fibers and the digestive tract. A diffuse interstitial fibrosis of the myocardium results and may lead to heart failure and death. The inflammatory lesions in the digestive tract that are seen in the esophagus and colon produce considerable dilatation. Chagas' disease has not been an important disease in the United States; most cases have been imported, although there are a few reports of endogenous disease in the southern United States.

375. The answer is a. (*Brooks, pp 575–580. Levinson, pp 321–323. Murray—2002, pp 714–715. Ryan, p 712.*) The febrile paroxysms of *Plasmodium malariae* malaria occur at 72-hour intervals; those of *P. falciparum* and *P. vivax* malaria occur every 48 hours. The paroxysms usually last 8 to 12 hours with *P. vivax* malaria but can last 16 to 36 hours with *P. falciparum* disease. In *P. vivax*, *Plasmodium ovale*, and *P. malariae* infections, all stages of development of the organisms can be seen in the peripheral blood; in malignant tertian (*P. falciparum*) infections, only early ring stages and gametocytes are usually found.

376. The answer is a. (*Brooks, pp 592–593. Levinson, pp 340–341. Murray—2002, pp 746–747. Ryan, pp 807–808.*) The Chinese liver fluke, *C. sinensis*, is a parasite of humans that is found in Japan, China, Korea, Taiwan, and Indochina. Humans usually are infected by eating uncooked fish. The worms invade bile ducts and produce destruction of liver parenchyma. Anemia, jaundice, weakness, weight loss, and tachycardia may follow. Treatment is likely to be ineffectual in heavy infections, but chloroquine can destroy some of the worms.

377. The answer is d. *(Brooks, pp 592–593. Levinson, pp 340–341. Murray—2002, pp 746–747. Ryan, pp 807–808.)* The life cycle of *C. sinensis* is similar to that of other trematodes. A mollusk is characteristically the first intermediate host of trematodes. For *C. sinensis*, snails perform this role.

378. The answer is b. *(Brooks, pp 575–580. Levinson, pp 321–323. Murray—2002, pp 715–716. Ryan, pp 711–722.)* The case history presented in the question is characteristic of infection with *P. falciparum*, the causative agent of malignant tertian malaria. The long duration of the febrile stage rules out other forms of malaria. The presence of ringlike young trophozoites and crescent-like mature gametocytes—as represented in the illustration below—as well as the absence of schizonts is diagnostic of *P. falciparum* malaria.

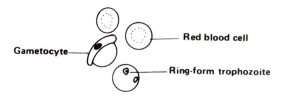

379. The answer is b. *(Brooks, p 555. Levinson, pp 324–325. Murray—2002, pp 664, 669–671. Ryan, pp 685–689.)* Both methenamine-silver and toluidine blue stain pneumocysts nonspecifically. These preparations are difficult to read because background material may nonspecifically stain black or blue. *P. carinii* cannot be routinely cultured from human specimens. Both IFA and DFA tests are FDA-approved and available for detection of *P. carinii*. The advantage of DFA is that it is quicker (45 to 60 minutes versus 3 hours) and there is less nonspecific fluorescence observed in the preparation. Recent evidence suggests that *Pneumocystis* is a fungus.

380. The answer is e. (*Brooks, pp 563–564. Levinson, p 320. Murray—2002, pp 703–704. Ryan, pp 742–745.*) *T. vaginalis* is the only protozoan listed where the trophozoite is the diagnostic and infective stage that feeds on the mucosal surface of the vagina (bacteria and leukocytes). The troph possesses a short, undulating membrane (one-half of the body) and four anterior flagella. No cyst stage exists. A persistent vaginitis with a frothy and foul-smelling discharge with burning, itching, and increased frequency of urination is common. Three to six million women in the United States are infected annually, while males are usually asymptomatic. Wet mounts examined in the laboratory reveal trophozites with rapid, jerky, and nondirectional motion.

381. The answer is a. (*Brooks, p 594. Levinson, pp 335–336. Murray—2002, pp 759–760. Ryan, pp 799–801.*) *E. granulosis* causes hydatid disease. The definitive hosts are dogs. Sheep, cattle, and humans are intermediate hosts. The adult tapeworm does not occur in humans. In the herbivores (infected by grazing where eggs have been deposited by carnivore feces), the eggs hatch and release hexacanths. These penetrate the gut and pass to other tissues (liver, viscera, muscle, and brain). Humans are only infected from dog feces and develop hydatid cysts, as described for herbivores. Diarrhea, therefore, does not occur with *E. granulosis* human infections, whereas the other four choices can routinely present with diarrhea.

382. The answer is e. (*Brooks, p 555. Levinson, pp 324–325. Murray—2002, pp 664, 669–671. Ryan, pp 685–689.*) One of the multiple criteria for classification of AIDS is the development of *P. carinii* pneumonia (PCP). *Pneumocystis* is a fungus formerly thought to be a parasite that was classified with the sporozoa. PCP may also be seen in patients with congenital or other acquired cellular immune dysfunction. Most patients with AIDS are given prophylactic aerosolized pentamidine or TMP-SXT for PCP. PCP is easily diagnosed in respiratory secretions by a direct fluorescent antibody test. Both the microsporidia and *Cryptosporidium* are intestinal parasites that also infect patients with AIDS, but these microorganisms cause protracted diarrhea. Both *Blastocystis* and *Blastomyces* are yeasts and should not be confused with *Pneumocystis* or each other.

383. The answer is c. (*Brooks, pp 594–595. Levinson, p 335. Murray—2002, pp 757–758. Ryan, pp 797–798.*) Consumption of raw fish causes endemic diphyllobothriasis in Scandinavia and the Baltic countries. While most people do not become ill, a small percentage (2%) develop vitamin B_{12} deficiency anemia. The adult fish tapeworm has an affinity for vitamin B_{12} and may induce a serious megaloblastic anemia. Parvovirus B19 causes acute hemolytic anemia primarily in immunosuppressed patients. *Yersinia* infection is common in Scandinavia but is not fish-borne and does not cause anemia. The larval stage of *T. solium* is called *cysticercus*. Humans usually acquire cysticercosis by ingestion of food and water contaminated by infected human feces.

384. The answer is e. *(Brooks, p 585. Levinson, pp 347–348. Murray— 2002, pp 734–736. Ryan, pp 763, 774–777.)* Strongyloidiasis may be observed in three phases: cutaneous, pulmonary, and intestinal. The pulmonary presentation of *Strongyloides* in patients with AIDS is the most common. Often, all body fluids will contain larvae. Prognosis is poor. *Necator* must be distinguished from *Strongyloides* by microscopy. Gross appearances are similar.

385. The answer is e. *(Brooks, p 303. Levinson, pp 157, 162, 164. Murray, pp 405, 777.)* *P. humanus* (head or body louse) and *Phthirus pubis* (crab louse) are wingless parasites exclusively affecting humans. Lice are important not only for the itching and discomfort they cause but also for the diseases they transmit. These disorders include epidemic typhus, relapsing fever, and trench fever. There is no evidence that lice secrete toxins.

386. The answer is c. *(Brooks, pp 575–580. Levinson, pp 321–323. Murray—2002, pp 715–716. Ryan, pp 711–722.)* Prophylaxis for malaria should be considered whenever a person is traveling in a malaria-endemic area. Drugs consist of mefloquine or chloroquine and Fansidar. Other control measures such as draining swamps, protective clothing and netting, and insect repellents are also effective. There is no currently available vaccine for malaria.

387. The answer is c. *(Murray, pp 770–771. Ryan, p 902.)* *Sarcoptes scabiei* is a small mite that burrows into human skin. Itching is significant, and a vesicular eruption, which often becomes secondarily infected with bacteria, develops. Diagnosis is made by microscopic detection of the mites. Gamma benzene hexachloride (Kwell), a topical insecticide, is an effective treatment for scabies. A number of etiologic agents have been proposed for Kawasaki's disease (KD), among them mites, but there is no evidence that mites either cause or are vectors of KD.

388. The answer is d. (*Brooks, pp 570–573. Levinson, pp 315–318. Murray—2002, pp 698–700. Ryan, pp 733–738.*) Of the intestinal amebas, *Entamoeba hartmanni*, *Entamoeba coli*, *Entamoeba polecki*, and *Entamoeba nana* are considered nonpathogenic. *E. histolytica* is distinctively characterized by its pathogenic potential for humans, although infection with this protozoan is commonly asymptomatic (causing "healthy carriers"). Symptomatic amebiasis and dysentery occur when the trophozoites invade the intestinal wall and produce ulceration and diarrhea. Peritonitis can occur, with the liver the most common site of extraintestinal disease. The life cycle of the ameba is simple by comparison. There is encystment of the troph, followed by excystation in the ileocecal region. The trophs multiply and become established in the cecum, where encystation takes place and results in abundant amebas, cysts, and trophozoites. Infection is spread by the cysts, which can remain for weeks or months in appropriately moist surroundings.

389. The answer is e. (*Brooks, pp 588–592. Levinson, pp 338–340. Murray—2002, pp 750–752. Ryan, pp 803, 808–813.*) Although the chronic stage of proliferation within tissues is distinctive in the different forms of schistosomiasis, a granulomatous reaction to the eggs and chemical products of the schistosome occurs in all forms of the disease. *S. haematobium* commonly involves the distal bowel and the bladder, as well as the prostate gland and seminal vesicles. Bladder calcification and cancer may ensue. *S. mansoni* affects the large bowel and the liver; presinusoidal portal hypertension, splenomegaly, and esophageal varices may be complications. Pulmonary hypertension, often fatal, may be seen with *S. mansoni* and *S. japonicum* disease. Eggs may be found in an unstained specimen of rectal mucosa or in stool. Urine microscopy and liver biopsy, when warranted, often prove positive. Schistosomiasis is best prevented by the elimination of the parasite in snails before human infection occurs.

390. The answer is d. (*Brooks, pp 290–291. Levinson, pp 155–157. Murray—2002, pp 384–390, 772–773. Ryan, pp 434–437.*) In the United States, *B. burgdorferi*, the causative agent of Lyme disease, has two principal vectors: *I. scapularis* in the eastern and midwestern United States and *I. pacificus* in the western United States. The ticks are tiny and can easily be missed. Fortunately, relatively few people who are bitten by ticks develop Lyme disease. Lyme disease, usually with joint involvement, is also seen in veterinary patients such as dogs, cats, and horses. White-tailed deer and small rodents are an important reservoir for these ticks. *B. burgdorferi* has been isolated from mosquitoes and *Dermacentor* and *Amblyomma* ticks as well as from several *Ixodes* species. However, the isolation of the bacterium from these ticks is not sufficient evidence to indicate that they transmit the disease to humans.

391. The answer is b. (*Brooks, p 585. Levinson, p 349. Murray—2002, pp 737–739. Ryan, pp 695–779, 784–785.*) *W. bancrofti* is the cause of bancroftian filariasis or filarial elephantiasis. Control of the mosquito vectors (culex, anopheles, and Aedes) is the most significant mechanism to control human infections. A disease of the tropics and subtropics, adults live in the lymphatics of a host and cause lymph blockage of the feet, arms, genitals, and breasts. Enlargement of the affected body part (elephantiasis) can then occur. Babesiosis is caused by tick-borne *Babesia microti*. Leishmaniasis is spread by a sand fly (Phlebotomus) vector. Guinea worms (*Dracunculus medinensis*) has an aquatic life cycle involving copepods (water fleas). Dog tapeworms would routinely be transmitted by fecal contamination.

392–395. The answers are 392-e, 393-a, 394-d, 395-c. (*Brooks, pp 591–593. Levinson, pp 338–342. Murray—2002, pp 774–753. Ryan, pp 803, 809–813.*) The life cycle of the medically important trematodes (or flukes) involves a sexual cycle in humans and an asexual cycle in snails. The schistosomes can penetrate the skin, whereas *Clonorchis* and *Paragonimus* are ingested, usually in fish or seafood. These flukes can be easily differentiated morphologically by the appearance of the egg. Schistosome eggs have an identifiable spine, and both *Clonorchis* and *Paragonimus* eggs are operculated; that is, they have what appears to be a cover that opens. Serological tests are not useful. Many patients with schistosomiasis are asymptomatic, but disease may become chronic, resulting in malaise, diarrhea, and hepatosplenomegaly (an enlarged liver and spleen). *Clonorchis* infection usually causes upper abdominal pain but can also cause biliary tract fibrosis. Paragonimiasis is characterized by a cough, often with bloody sputum, and pneumonia. Praziquantel is the treatment of choice for these flukes.

396–399. The answers are 396-c, 397-e, 398-a, 399-b. (*Brooks, pp 562–563, 564, 585, 590. Levinson, pp 315–316, 318–319, 346–348. Murray— 2002, pp 698–703, 730–731, 734–736. Ryan, pp 695–696, 733–738, 745–748, 769–771, 774–777.*) It is not uncommon that repeated stool specimens do not reveal the suspected parasite. Also, microscopic analysis of stool may not reveal parasite load when such data are necessary. For these reasons, other techniques are available to identify parasites as well as to quantitate them.

During sigmoidoscopy, a curette or suction device may be used to scrape or aspirate material from the mucosal surface. Cotton swabs should not be used. A direct mount of this material should immediately be examined for *E. histolytica* trophozoites, and then a permanent stain made for subsequent examination.

The Baermann technique may be helpful in recovering *Strongyloides* larvae. Essentially, fecal material is placed on damp gauze on the top of a glass funnel that is three-quarters filled with water. The larvae migrate through the damp gauze and into the water. The water may then be centrifuged to concentrate the *Strongyloides*.

Worm burdens may be estimated by a number of microscopic methods. While not often done, such procedures may provide data on the extent of infection or the efficacy of treatment of hookworms, *Ascaris*, or *Trichuris*. Thirty thousand *Trichuris* eggs per gram, 2000 to 5000 hookworm eggs per gram, and 1 *Ascaris* egg are clinically significant and suggest a heavy worm burden.

The diagnosis of giardiasis is usually made by detecting trophozoites and cysts of *G. lamblia* in consecutive fecal specimens. Alternatively, a gelatin capsule on a string (enterotest) can be swallowed, passed to the duodenum, and then retrieved after four hours. The string is then examined for *Giardia*. A recent innovation is the introduction of an enzyme immunoassay (EIA) for *G. lamblia*. The EIA is more sensitive than microscopy, can be performed on a single stool specimen, and does not depend on the presence of entire trophozoites and cysts. A cellophane tape swab is used to trap pinworms crawling out of the anus during the night. The tape is then examined microscopically for *Enterobius*.

400–404. The answers are 400-c, 401-d, 402-a, 403-b, 404-e. (*Brooks, pp 562–563, 582–584, 587–590, 593–594. Levinson, pp 318–319, 323–324, 332–335, 338–340, 351–352. Murray—2002, pp 701–703,*

717–720, 731–732, 750–752, 754–757. Ryan, pp 695–696, 723–727, 746–748, 779–784, 809–813.) All the diseases listed in the question have significant epidemiologic and clinical features. Toxoplasmosis, for example, is generally a mild, self-limiting disease; however, severe fetal disease is possible if pregnant women ingest *Toxoplasma* oocysts. Consumption of uncooked meat may result in either an acute toxoplasmosis or a chronic toxoplasmosis that is associated with serious eye disease. Most adults have antibody titers to *Toxoplasma* and thus would have a positive Sabin-Feldman dye test.

Trichinosis most often is caused by ingestion of contaminated pork products. However, eating undercooked bear, walrus, raccoon, or possum meat also may cause this disease. Symptoms of trichinosis include muscle soreness and swollen eyes.

Although giardiasis has been classically associated with travel in Russia, especially St. Petersburg (Leningrad), many cases of giardiasis caused by contaminated water have been reported in the United States as well. Diagnosis is made by detecting cysts in the stool. In some cases, diagnosis may be very difficult because of the relatively small number of cysts present. Alternatively, an enzyme immunoassay may be used to detect *Giardia* antigen in fecal samples.

Schistosomiasis is a worldwide public health problem. Control of this disease entails the elimination of the intermediate host snail and removal of streamside vegetation. Abdominal pain is a symptom of schistosomiasis.

Visceral larva migrans is an occupational disease of people who are in close contact with dogs and cats. The disease is caused by the nematodes *Toxocara canis* (dogs) and *Toxocara cati* (cats) and has been recognized in young children who have close contact with pets or who eat dirt. Symptoms include skin rash, eosinophilia, and hepatosplenomegaly.

405–409. The answers are 405-e, 406-a, 407-d, 408-c, 409-b. (*Brooks, pp 562–564, 580–581, 590–593. Levinson, pp 318–320, 330, 341, 349. Murray—2002, pp 701–704, 716–717, 736–737, 747–749. Ryan, pp 695–696, 741–745, 746–748, 779, 781–784, 803, 805–807.*) T. vaginalis, an odd-looking protozoan, moves with a jerky, almost darting motion. Trichomoniasis, a bothersome vaginal infection, can be diagnosed by observing this organism in a wet mount of vaginal secretions. It may be washed out in the urine as well. *T. vaginalis* can be grown in special media, and there are now several products available for direct detection of the organism.

Trichinella spiralis causes trichinosis, a parasitic disease that is usually mild and results in muscle pain and a mild febrile illness. However, fulminant fatal cases have been described. Humans, who are accidental hosts, become infected by ingesting cysts that are in the muscle of animals. Most infections still come from pork, although regulations on pig feeding have markedly reduced the incidence. Laboratory diagnosis is by serology or demonstration of the larvae in the muscle tissue.

Paragonimus westermani is a lung fluke. This trematode infects lung tissue and is seen not only in sputum but also in feces because infected patients swallow respiratory secretions. Paragonimiasis is contracted by ingesting the metacercariae that are encysted in crabs or crayfish.

Giardia infection may be difficult to diagnose by stool examination, as patients may shed the cysts intermittently. When symptoms persist and the stool examination is negative, then duodenal contents may be sampled directly with the enterotest. The patient swallows a gelatin capsule that contains a coiled string. The other end is attached to the patient's face. The gelatin capsule dissolves, and *Giardia* organisms, if present, adhere to the string within a four-hour period. The string is retrieved and examined microscopically. Alternatively, an enzymatic immunoassay can detect *Giardia* antigen directly in a single specimen of feces.

Babesia is a sporozoan parasite transmitted by the bite of *I. scapularis,* the same tick that carries *B. burgdorferi.* Reproduction of this parasite occurs in erythrocytes and may resemble *Plasmodium* species when blood smears are examined. *Babesia* is endemic in the northeastern United States, particularly in the islands of Massachusetts. Laboratory diagnosis is made by examining blood smears for this parasite or by detection of specific antibody. Babesiosis clinically resembles malaria.

Immunology

Questions

DIRECTIONS: Each question below contains four or more suggested responses. Select the **one best** response to each question.

Item 410–413

Hypersensitivity reactions are exaggerated or inappropriate immune responses that can sometimes result in damage to the host instead of providing protection. The four main types are represented below:

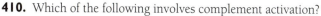

410. Which of the following involves complement activation?
a. 1
b. 2
c. 3
d. 4
e. 1 and 2
f. 1 and 3
g. 1 and 4
h. 2 and 3

411. After playing in the bushes during a camping trip, a 7-year-old girl complains of intense itching and blistering of the hands, arms, and legs. Which of the following is the most likely condition and which is the representative hypersensitivity diagram, respectively, from those presented above?

a. Contact dermatitis and 2
b. Contact dermatitis and 3
c. Contact dermatitis and 4
d. Arthrus reaction and 1
e. Arthrus reaction and 2
f. Arthrus reaction and 3

412. Skin testing is useful in the diagnosis of which one of the following?

a. 1 and 2
b. 1 and 3
c. 1 and 4
d. 2, 3, and 4

413. Rh disease and Goodpasture's syndrome are best represented by which one of the following?

a. 1 and 2
b. 2 and 3
c. 2 and 4
d. 2 only
e. 3 only

Item 414–415

A 7-month-old male infant presented to the emergency department with severe middle ear and upper respiratory tract infections, which responded promptly to antibiotics. Two months later he was again admitted, this time with *Streptococcus pneumoniae* pneumonia. After several more episodes of bacterial infections, genetic testing was done and revealed the presence of a defective B cell tyrosine kinase gene (btk gene or X-LA gene). In addition, physical exam detected very small tonsils.

414. Which of the following is the most likely diagnosis?

a. Ataxia telangiectasia
b. Bruton's agammaglobulinemia
c. Chronic granulomatous disease
d. Late (C5, C6, C7, C8, C9) complement deficiency
e. Thymic aplasia (DiGeorge's syndrome)

415. Which of the following pathogens will present the most serious threat to this child?

a. *Chlamydia trachomatis*
b. Measles virus
c. *Mycobacterium tuberculosis*
d. Varicella-zoster virus (VZV)

416. Megakaryocytes are minimally immunoresponsive; such cells give rise to which of the following?

a. B lymphocytes
b. Cytokines
c. Interleukins
d. Platelets
e. T lymphocytes

417. One of the most remarkable aspects of the human immune system is its diversity, that is, the ability to recognize a wide range of antigens and to mount a specific antibody response. This is called *clonal selection*. At the cellular level, which of the following are primarily responsible for such specificity?

a. Cytotoxic T cells
b. Hypervariable regions in domains of B cells
c. Memory cells
d. Specific T cell receptors
e. The major histocompatibility complex

418. A young girl has had repeated infections with *Candida albicans* and respiratory viruses since she was three months old. As part of the clinical evaluation of her immune status, her responses to routine immunization procedures should be tested. In this evaluation, the use of which of the following vaccines is contraindicated?

a. BCG
b. *Bordetella pertussis* vaccine
c. Diphtheria toxoid
d. Inactivated polio
e. Tetanus toxoid

419. A latent, measles-like viral infection and, presumably, a defect in cellular immunity is associated with which of the following diseases?

a. Creutzfeldt-Jakob disease
b. Epstein-Barr virus (EBV) infection
c. Multiple sclerosis (MS)
d. Progressive multifocal leukoencephalopathy (PML)
e. Subacute sclerosing panencephalitis (SSPE)

420. In humans, two closely linked genetic loci, each made up of two alleles, compose the histocompatibility locus A (HL-A). Paired first and second locus antigens are called *haplotypes*. The HL-A haplotypes (separated by a semicolon) of a child's parents are given below:

Father 3,25;7,12
Mother 1,3;8,9

   Assuming that no crossover events have occurred, the child's histotype could be which of the following?

a. 1,3;7,8
b. 7,12;1,3
c. 3,3;7,9
d. 1,25;7,12
e. 3,25;7,12

421. The following graph shows the sequential alteration in the type and amount of antibody produced after an immunization. (Inoculation of antigen occurs at two different times, as indicated by the arrows.) Curve A and curve B each represent a distinct type of antibody. The class of immunoglobulin represented by curve B has which of the following characteristics?

a. A composition of four peptide chains connected by disulfide links
b. A symmetric dipeptide
c. An appearance in neonates at approximately the third month of life
d. An estimated molecular weight of 150,000
e. The human ABO isoagglutinin

422. Which of the statements about the precipitin curve shown below is true?

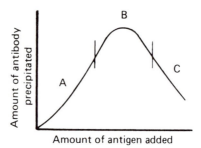

a. A solution in zone A would be expected to have unreacted precipitable antigen in the supernatant
b. A solution in zone C would be expected to have both antigen and antibody in excess
c. A solution in zone C would be expected to have an excess of antibody in the supernatant
d. In a multispecific system, a solution in zone B would have only an excess of antigen in the supernatant
e. In a monospecific system, a solution in zone B would contain only reacted antibody and antigen

423. A widely used method for detecting either antigen or antibody in body fluids is known as ELISA (enzyme-linked immunosorbent assay). The figure below demonstrates an ELISA for detection of antigen. One of the problems with ELISA is nonspecific reactivity due to nonspecific antibody present in the reaction. Of the four steps depicted, A, B, C, and D, which one may be the major cause of nonspecificity?

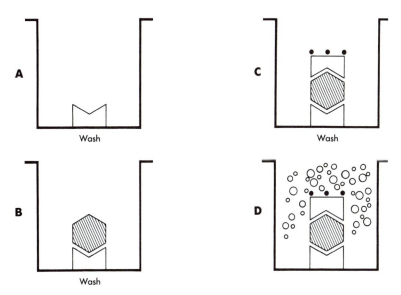

Double antibody sandwich method of EIA for assay of antigen. **A,** antibody is adsorbed to surface. **B,** test solution containing antigen is added. **C,** enzyme-labeled specific antibody is added. **D,** enzyme substrate is added.

a. A
b. B
c. C
d. D

424. An Ouchterlony gel diffusion plate shows the reaction of a polyspe-cific serum against several antigen preparations. The center well in Figure 1 contains polyspecific antiserum, first bleed; the center well in Figure 2 contains polyspecific antiserum, second bleed; NS is normal saline. In this situation, cross-reaction can be recognized between antigen X and which of the following antigens?

Figure 1   Figure 2

a. A
b. B
c. C
d. D
e. E

425. A patient presents with marked susceptibility to opportunistic infec-tions with bacteria such as *Escherichia coli* and *Staphylococcus aureus,* and *Aspergillus.* Exam findings reveal granulomatous abscesses in the lungs. Biochemical analysis reveals the deficiency of the central enzyme in the res-piratory burst pathway via an inability to reduce nitroblue tetrazolium (NBT) dye. After further testing, a diagnosis of chronic granulomatous dis-ease is rendered. The deficient enzyme and reaction are represented by which of the following?

a. $NADPH + 2O_2$ NADPH oxidase $\longrightarrow NADP^+ + 2O_2^- + H^+$

b. $2O_2^- + 2H^+$ Superoxide dismutase $\longrightarrow H_2O_2 + O_2$

c. $H_2O_2 + Cl^-$ Myelopeoxidase $\longrightarrow H_2O + OCl^-$

d. $\frac{1}{2}O_2 + $ arginine   NO synthase $\longrightarrow NO + $ citrulline

e. $2H^+ + 2e^- + \frac{1}{2}O_2$ Oxidase $\longrightarrow H_2O$

f. $2H_2O_2$ Catalase $\longrightarrow 2H_2O + O_2$

426. Chromosomal analysis of a patient suffering from a lymphoma revealed the following result:

(*Reproduced, with permission, from Parslow TG et al. Medical Immunology, 10e. New York: McGraw-Hill, 2001, 113.*)

According to the above figure, the patient has which of the following?
a. Anaplastic large cell lymphoma
b. Burkitt's lymphoma
c. Follicular lymphoma
d. Mantle cell lymphoma

427. Which statement best applies to the diagram below?

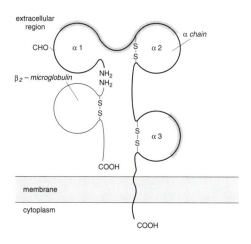

(Modified, with permission, from Parslow TG et al. Medical Immunology, 10e. New York: McGraw-Hill, 2001, 85.)

a. Depicts the cell-membrane MHC product associated with narcolepsy
b. Essential for the transplacental passage of antibody
c. Found on memory T and B lymphocytes
d. Present on macrophages but not neutrophils
e. Represents the secretory component associated with IgA
f. Required for recognition of processed antigen by T_H1 and T_H2 lymphocytes

428. A 19-year-old college student develops a rash. She works part-time in a pediatric AIDS clinic. Her blood is drawn and tested for specific antibody to the chickenpox virus (varicella-zoster). Which of the following antibody classes would you expect to find if she is immune to chickenpox?

a. IgG
b. IgA
c. IgM
d. IgD
e. IgE

Questions 429–431

429. A 34-year-old male patient visits a physician with complaints of fatigue, weight loss, night sweats, and "swollen glands." The physician also observes that he has an oral yeast infection. Which of the following tests would most likely reveal the cause of his problems?
a. A human T-lymphotropic virus type I (HTLV-I) test
b. A test for *C. albicans*
c. A test for CD8 lymphocytes
d. A test for infectious mononucleosis
e. An HIV ELISA test

430. The figure below demonstrates a western blot for HIV. Based on these results, and assuming a repeatedly reactive ELISA HIV screening test, which of the following is your best course of action?

gp 160

gp 120

p 66

p 51

gp 41

p 24

p 17

a. Consider anti-HIV therapy
b. Inform the patient that the test is falsely positive
c. Order an HIV RNA test
d. Repeat the test immediately
e. Wait six weeks and repeat the test

431. A second patient makes an appointment. This patient, a 30-year-old male, requests a routine HIV test. The HIV ELISA was weakly positive and is repeated with the same results. The western blot result is as shown in the preceding figure. The patient denies any risk factors for HIV. Which of the following is the most likely cause of a falsely positive HIV test?

a. A recent flu shot
b. A yeast infection
c. Naturally occurring HIV antibody
d. Test cross-reactivity with Epstein-Barr virus
e. Test cross-reactivity with HTLV

432. Patients with C5 through C9 complement deficiencies are most likely to be susceptible to which of the following infections?

a. AIDS
b. Giardiasis
c. Histoplasmosis
d. Meningococcal infection
e. Pneumococcal infection

433. As part of the management of a 28-year-old male with acute onset of Crohn's disease of the small bowel, you decide to treat him with a new cocktail of mouse-human chimeric antibodies to reduce his intestinal inflammation and cachexia. To what set of proteins may these antibodies be directed?

a. IL-1, IL-2, IL-3
b. IL-2, IL-12, TNF-α
c. IL-2, TGF-β, TNF-α
d. IL-1, IL-6, TNF-α
e. IL-2, IL-3, IL-12

434. Immunity may be innate or acquired. Which of the following best describes acquired immunity?

a. Complement cascade
b. Increase in C-reactive protein (CRP)
c. Inflammatory response
d. Maternal transfer of antibody
e. Presence of natural killer (NK) cells

435. A 35-year-old male patient presents with numerous subcutaneous hemorrhages. History and physical exam reveal that he has been taking sedormid (a sedative) for the past week. Laboratory tests indicate normal hemoglobin and white blood cell levels with significant thrombocytopenia (very low platelet count). You suspect that he has developed a drug-induced type II hypersensitivity reaction. This reaction may occur if the drug does which of the following?

a. Activates T cytotoxic cells
b. Acts as a hapten
c. Induces mast cell degranulation releasing mediators such as histamine, leukotrienes, and prostaglandins
d. Induces oxygen radical production through the respiratory burst pathway
e. Persists in macrophages

436. The major role of T cells in the immune response includes which one of the following?

a. Complement fixation
b. Phagocytosis
c. Production of antibodies
d. Recognition of epitopes presented with major histocompatibility complex molecules on all surfaces

437. Which of the following statements is true of immunoglobulins?

a. Digestion of an IgG antibody molecule with papain yields two F(ab) arms, which are unable to agglutinate or precipitate antigen, by cleaving the antibody unit on the C terminus side of the sulfhydral bridge binding the heavy chain
b. In humans, there are approximately twice as many Ig molecules with κ and λ light chains
c. In the three-dimensional structure of Ig, there is little if any flexibility in the hinge region between the Fc and two F(ab) portions
d. Normally, IgG makes up 20% of the antibody concentration and migrates in the gamma globulin fraction of serum protein separation
e. Pepsin digestion of an IgG molecule cleaves the antibody unit on the N-terminus side of the sulfhydryl bridge binding the heavy chains
f. The two arms of an antibody molecule are different in that they recognize different epitopes

438. A 31-year-old male patient complains of fatigue, yeast infection in his mouth, and enlarged lymph nodes under his arms. He said that he was involved in "high-risk" behavior six years ago while on a trip to eastern and southern Africa. He also indicated that his "HIV test" was negative. Which one of the following options would be most appropriate?

a.   Initiate treatment for HIV disease
b.   Order a test for human T cell leukemia virus (HTLV)
c.   Order an HIV-1 RNA PCR
d.   Order an HIV test that would include antibodies to HIV-1 and HIV-2
e.   Repeat the test for HIV-1

439. A laboratory analysis report of a specific fraction of a patient's lymphocytes indicates the following:

HLA, B, and C+, PHA+, CD3−, CD16+, CD11a/CD18+, CD56+, and in vitro blastogenesis with IL-12

What are the lymphocytes this set describes?

a.   B lymphocytes
b.   Cytotoxic T lymphocytes
c.   Natural killer cells
d.   T helper 1 subset
e.   T helper 2 subset

440. The complement system plays a key role in the host defense process. Which component of this system, listed below, is the most important in chemotaxis?

a.   C1q
b.   C3a
c.   C3b
d.   C4a
e.   C5a

441. A 7-year-old child presents to your clinic during flu season with a severe headache, sinus congestion, fever, sore throat, and cough. Respiratory secretions reveal detectable levels of the cytokine interferon. What is the mechanism of action of this cytokine?

a. Binds extracellular virus particles and prevents cellular adherence
b. Upregulates the synthesis of secretory proteins that bind and inhibit the virus particles
c. Disrupts viral and cellular protein synthesis, leading to cellular apoptosis
d. Inhibits viral protein synthesis by degrading viral mRNA
e. Downregulates cellular protein synthesis, leading to decreased levels of viral receptors on the cytoplasmic membrane

442. Survival of allografts is increased by choosing donors with few major histocompatibility complex (MHC) mismatches with recipients and by use of immunosuppression in recipients. Which one of the following procedures might be a useful measure of immunosuppression?

a. Administration of corticosteroids to recipient
b. Administration of immunoglobulin to recipient
c. Destruction of donor B cells
d. Destruction of donor T cells
e. Lymphoid irradiation of donor

443. Relative to the primary immunological response, secondary and later booster responses to a given hapten-protein complex can be associated with which one of the following?

a. Antibodies that are less efficient in preventing specific disease
b. Decreased antibody avidity for the original hapten-protein complex
c. Increased antibody affinity for the hapten
d. Lower titers of antibody
e. Maintenance of the same subclass, or idiotype, of antibody produced

444. You are managing a 3-year-old female patient with a fever of unknown origin. Her serum is tested for antibodies against *Haemophilus influenzae*. A precipitation test conducted by the clinical laboratory yields the following results:

Serum (Antibody) Dilutions

Undiluted serum	1:2	1:4	1:8	1:16	1:32	1:64	1:128	1:256
−	+	+	+	+	+	+	−	−

From this data, which of the following can be concluded?

a. Postzone occurs at undiluted 1:2; zone of equivalence occurs at 1:2–1:64; and prozone occurs at 1:128
b. The negative reactions at 1:128 and 1:126 are false negatives
c. The patient has antibodies against *H. influenzae*, the titer is 64, and the dilution 1:64
d. The patient has antibodies against *H. influenzae*, the dilution is 64, and the titer 1:64
e. The patient does not have antibodies against *H. influenzae* since the reaction is negative with undiluted serum
f. The patient should be immunized against *H. influenzae*
g. The test needs to be repeated because the results cannot be interpreted

445. IgA antibody is the first line of defense against infections at the mucous membrane. It is usually an early specific antibody. Which of the following statements regarding IgA is true?

a. Complement fixation tests for IgA antibody will be positive if specific IgA antibody is present
b. IgA can be destroyed by bacterial proteases
c. IgA is absent in colostrum
d. IgA is not found in saliva; therefore, an IgA diagnostic test on saliva would have no value
e. IgA is a small molecule with a molecular weight of 30,000 kDa

446. Complement is a series of important host proteins that provide protection from invasion by foreign microorganisms. Which one of the following statements best describes complement?

a. Complement inhibits phagocytosis
b. Complement is activated by IgE antibody classes
c. Complement plays a minor role in the inflammatory response
d. Complement protects the host from pneumococcal infection through C1, C2, and C4
e. Microorganisms agglutinate in the presence of complement but do not lyse

Item 447–451

The following five questions relate to immunoglobulins, IgG, A, M, D, and E.

447. Which immunoglobulin has no known function, is found in the serum in low concentrations, and is present on the surface of B lymphocytes (may function as an antigen receptor)?

a. IgG
b. IgA
c. IgM
d. IgD
e. IgE

448. Present as a monomer on B cell surfaces but as a pentamer in serum, which of the following is the immunoglobulin that is initially seen in the primary immune response?

a. IgG
b. IgA
c. IgM
d. IgD
e. IgE

449. Which immunoglobulin mediates immediate hypersensitivity and is involved in immune response to parasitic infections?

a. IgG
b. IgA
c. IgM
d. IgD
e. IgE

450. Which immunoglobulin is the primary antibody in saliva, tears, and intestinal and genital secretions?

a. IgG
b. IgA
c. IgM
d. IgD
e. IgE

451. With four subclasses, which immunoglobulin is the predominant antibody in the secondary immune response?

a. IgG
b. IgA
c. IgM
d. IgD
e. IgE

Questions 452–456

452. IgM antibody (1:200) to *Borrelia burgdorferi* is associated with which one of the following?

a. Acute Lyme disease
b. Fifth disease
c. Possible hepatitis B infection
d. Possible subacute sclerosing panencephalitis (SSPE)
e. Susceptibility to chickenpox

453. Elevated IgG and IgM antibody titers to Parvovirus suggest a diagnosis of which one of the following?

a. Acute Lyme disease
b. Fifth disease
c. Possible hepatitis B infection
d. Possible subacute sclerosing panencephalitis (SSPE)
e. Susceptibility to chickenpox

454. A negative varicella antibody titer in a young woman signifies which one of the following?

a. Acute Lyme disease
b. Fifth disease
c. Possible hepatitis B infection
d. Possible subacute sclerosing panencephalitis (SSPE)
e. Susceptibility to chickenpox

455. A patient has an increased antibody titer to delta agent. You would most likely suspect which one of the following?

a. Acute Lyme disease
b. Fifth disease
c. Possible hepatitis B infection
d. Possible subacute sclerosing panencephalitis (SSPE)
e. Susceptibility to chickenpox

456. A patient with neurological problems has an elevated cerebrospinal fluid (CSF) antibody titer to measles virus. You would most likely suspect which one of the following?

a. Acute Lyme disease
b. Fifth disease
c. Possible hepatitis B infection
d. Possible subacute sclerosing panencephalitis (SSPE)
e. Susceptibility to chickenpox

Questions 457–461

Certain diseases are associated with a level of immune dysfunction (humoral, cellular, or both).

457. Ataxia-telangiectasia usually is associated with which one of the following?

	Humoral	Cellular
a.	Normal	Normal
b.	Normal	Deficient
c.	Deficient	Normal
d.	Deficient	Deficient
e.	Elevated	Elevated

458. Infantile X-linked agammaglobulinemia (Bruton's disease) is usually associated with which one of the following?

	Humoral	Cellular
a.	Normal	Normal
b.	Normal	Deficient
c.	Deficient	Normal
d.	Deficient	Deficient
e.	Elevated	Elevated

459. Severe combined immunodeficiency (SCID) is usually associated with which one of the following?

	Humoral	Cellular
a.	Normal	Normal
b.	Normal	Deficient
c.	Deficient	Normal
d.	Deficient	Deficient
e.	Elevated	Elevated

460. Thymic hypoplasia (DiGeorge's syndrome) is usually associated with which one of the following?

	Humoral	**Cellular**
a.	Normal	Normal
b.	Normal	Deficient
c.	Deficient	Normal
d.	Deficient	Deficient
e.	Elevated	Elevated

461. Wiskott-Aldrich syndrome is usually associated with which one of the following?

	Humoral	**Cellular**
a.	Normal	Normal
b.	Normal	Deficient
c.	Deficient	Normal
d.	Deficient	Deficient
e.	Elevated	Elevated

Questions 462–465

462. An autograft is best described by which one of the following statements?

a. Transplant from one region of a person to another region
b. Transplant from one person to a genetically identical person
c. Transplant from one species to the same species
d. Transplant from one species to another species

463. An isograft is best described by which one of the following statements?

a. Transplant from one region of a person to another region
b. Transplant from one person to a genetically identical person
c. Transplant from one species to the same species
d. Transplant from one species to another species

464. An allograft is best described by which one of the following statements?

a. Transplant from one region of a person to another region
b. Transplant from one person to a genetically identical person
c. Transplant from one species to the same species
d. Transplant from one species to another species

465. A xenograft is best described by which one of the following statements?

a. Transplant from one region of a person to another region
b. Transplant from one person to a genetically identical person
c. Transplant from one species to the same species
d. Transplant from one species to another species

Item 466–468

Antigenic determinants on immunoglobulins are used to classify antibodies.

466. An isotype is characterized by which one of the following statements?

a. Determinant exposed after papain cleavage to an F(ab) fragment
b. Determinant from one clone of cells and probably located close to the antigen-binding site of the immunoglobulin
c. Determinant inherited in a Mendelian fashion and recognized by cross-immunization of individuals in a species
d. Heavy-chain determinant recognized by heterologous antisera
e. Species-specific carbohydrate determinant on the heavy chain

467. An allotype is characterized by which one of the following statements?

a. Determinant exposed after papain cleavage to an F(ab) fragment
b. Determinant from one clone of cells and probably located close to the antigen-binding site of the immunoglobulin
c. Determinant inherited in a Mendelian fashion and recognized by cross-immunization of individuals in a species
d. Heavy-chain determinant recognized by heterologous antisera
e. Species-specific carbohydrate determinant on the heavy chain

468. An idiotype is characterized by which one of the following statements?

a. Determinant exposed after papain cleavage to an F(ab')2 fragment
b. Determinant from one clone of cells and probably located close to the antigen-binding site of the immunoglobulin
c. Determinant inherited in a Mendelian fashion and recognized by cross-immunization of individuals in a species
d. Heavy-chain determinant recognized by heterologous antisera
e. Species-specific carbohydrate determinant on the heavy chain

469. A 30-year-old male presents to the emergency room with difficulty breathing and abdominal pain. Upon physical exam, you notice diffuse areas of nondependent, nonpitting swelling without pruritus, with predilection for the face, especially the perioral and periorbital areas. You also notice swelling in the mouth, pharynx, and larynx. Laboratory analysis of blood drawn from this patient indicates a complement problem. Which of the following is most likely?

a. High C1 and normal level of C1 esterase inhibitor
b. High C1 esterase inhibitor and low C4
c. Low C4 and high C2
d. High C4, C2, and C3
e. Low C1 esterase inhibitor and low C4

470. A 45-year-old businesswoman arrives in your office with vagus abdominal complaints. She has noticed melenic stool. Upon performing a sigmoidoscopy, you find a 4-cm mass in the upper colon. You immediately order a blood test for which of the following tumor markers?

a. Alpha-fetoprotein
b. Antitumor antibody
c. Antitumor light chains
d. Carcinoembryonic antigen
e. Human chorionic gonadotropin
f. Prostate-specific antigen

Item 471–472

An 18-year-old male heroin addict, who practices the sharing of needles at a "shooting gallery," is positive in the screening test for AIDS.

471. This patient is most likely to be immunodeficient because of which one of the following?

a. A genetic defect in chromosome 14
b. A low T helper lymphocyte count
c. An atrophied thymus
d. NADPH enzyme deficiency
e. Insufficient B cell maturation

472. Since a false positive is possible, the physician orders a confirmatory test. Which of the following best describes the standard confirmatory test and what this test checks for, respectively?

a. Complement fixation test; antibodies against the virus
b. Enzyme-linked immunosorbent assay; antigens of the virus
c. Radioimmunoassay; specific antibodies against the virus
d. Western blot; antigens of the virus
e. Western blot; specific antibodies against the virus

473. A pregnant 21-year-old Rh-negative female is about to deliver. The baby's father is determined to be Rh-positive. To reduce the chance for the development of hemolytic disease of the newborn, which of the following procedures would you order?

a. Administration of anti-Rh antibodies to the fetus postdelivery
b. Administration of anti-Rh antibodies to the mother postdelivery
c. Immediate blood transfusion of the suspected father
d. Immediate blood transfusion of the mother with Rh-positive blood
e. Infusion of immune serum globulin into the fetus
f. Intravenous infusion of the Rh antigen into the mother

Item 474–475

An 8-month-old male infant with a history of chronic diarrhea, otitis media, and several episodes of pneumonia presents to your clinic with gingivostomatitis (due to herpes simplex virus) and oral candidiasis (thrush). You immediately order an x-ray and a blood workup. X-ray and laboratory blood analysis reveal the absence of a thymic shadow and absence of B lymphocytes, respectively. History taken from the infant's mother reveals a rash evident at birth.

474. Which of the following diseases is most likely to be present in this infant?

a. Ataxia-telangiectasia
b. Bruton's agammaglobulinemia
c. Chediak-Higashi syndrome
d. Chronic granulomatous disease
e. Chronic mucocutaneous candidiasis
f. Hereditary angioedema
g. Severe combined immunodeficiency syndrome (SCID)
h. Thymic aplasia (DiGeorge's syndrome)
i. Wiskott-Aldrich syndrome

475. What is the best therapy for this infant?

a. Antifungal agents
b. Blood transfusion
c. Bone marrow transplant
d. IgG from pooled random donors
e. Immunization with attenuated vaccines

476. A 5-year-old child arrives at the emergency department minutes after being bitten by a black widow spider. You immediately inject gamma globulin in the form of an antivenom. This type of immunization is referred to as which of the following?

a. Artificial active immunization
b. Artificial passive immunization
c. Natural active immunization
d. Natural passive immunization
e. Adoptive immunization

477. A patient with an increased susceptibility to viral, fungal, and protozoa infection would be expected to have a deficiency in which of the following cell types?

a. B lymphocytes
b. Macrophages
c. Natural killer cells
d. Neutrophils
e. T lymphocytes

Item 478–479

Complement fixation (CF) testing is an important serological tool. One has to understand the conditions under which complement is bound and RBCs are lysed.

478. Anti-*Mycoplasma* antibody + complement + hemolysin-sensitized red blood cells (RBCs) + anti-RBC antibody results in which one of the following?

a. Complement is bound; RBCs are lysed
b. Complement is bound; RBCs are not lysed
c. Complement is not bound; RBCs are lysed
d. Complement is not bound; RBCs are not lysed
e. Complement is not bound; RBCs are agglutinated

479. Anti-*Mycoplasma* antibody + *Mycoplasma* antigen + complement + hemolysin-sensitized RBCs + anti-RBC antibody results in which one of the following?

a. Complement is bound; RBCs are lysed
b. Complement is bound; RBCs are not lysed
c. Complement is not bound; RBCs are lysed
d. Complement is not bound; RBCs are not lysed
e. Complement is not bound; RBCs are agglutinated

480. While walking through a field, a 28-year-old woman is accidentally stung by a bee. Within 10 minutes she has asthmatic-like symptoms. This type of hypersensitivity reaction can be correctly characterized by which of the following sequences of steps?

a. Allergen, chemical mediators, sensitization, allergen, IgE, symptoms
b. Allergen, IgE, sensitization, allergen, chemical mediators, symptoms
c. Allergen, sensitization, IgE, allergen, chemical mediators, symptoms
d. Sensitization, allergen, chemical mediators, allergen, IgE, symptoms
e. Sensitization, IgE, allergen, symptoms, allergen, chemical mediators

Item 481–485

Most, but not all, cases of hepatitis are caused by hepatitis A virus (HAV), hepatitis B virus (HBV), or non-A, non-B hepatitis virus (hepatitis C virus). While the laboratory diagnosis of HAV is usually accomplished by the detection of IgG and IgM antibodies to HAV, the diagnosis of HBV is more complex.

481. Finding IgG antibodies to core antigen, antibodies to e antigen, and antibodies to surface antigen reflects which of the following?

a. Acute infection (incubation period)
b. Acute infection (acute phase)
c. Postinfection (acute phase)
d. Immunization
e. HBV carrier state

482. Finding HBsAg positive and HBeAg positive reflects which of the following?

a. Acute infection (incubation period)
b. Acute infection (acute phase)
c. Postinfection (acute phase)
d. Immunization
e. HBV carrier state

483. Finding HBsAg positive, HBeAg positive, and IgM core antibody positive reflects which of the following?

a. Acute infection (incubation period)
b. Acute infection (acute phase)
c. Postinfection (acute phase)
d. Immunization
e. HBV carrier state

484. Finding HBsAg positive, no antibodies to HBsAg, and other tests variable reflects which of the following?

a. Acute infection (incubation period)
b. Acute infection (acute phase)
c. Postinfection (acute phase)
d. Immunization
e. HBV carrier state

485. Finding antibodies to HBsAg reflects which of the following?

a. Acute infection (incubation period)
b. Acute infection (acute phase)
c. Postinfection (acute phase)
d. Immunization
e. HBV carrier state

Item 486–490

There are a variety of immunologic tests available for the detection of both antigen and antibody.

486. Which of the following tests combines features of gel diffusion and immunoelectrophoresis and is applicable only to negatively charged antigens?

a. Coagglutination (COA)
b. Counterimmunoelectrophoresis (CIE)
c. Enzyme-linked immunosorbent assay (ELISA)
d. Latex agglutination (LA)
e. Radioimmunoassay (RIA)

487. Which of the following tests depends on the presence of protein Λ on certain strains of *S. aureus?*

a. Coagglutination (COA)
b. Counterimmunoelectrophoresis (CIE)
c. Enzyme-linked immunosorbent assay (ELISA)
d. Latex agglutination (LA)
e. Radioimmunoassay (RIA)

488. Which of the following tests involves the measurement of very small quantities through competition of radiolabeled and unlabeled antigen for the same limited amount of antibody?

a. Coagglutination (COA)
b. Counterimmunoelectrophoresis (CIE)
c. Enzyme-linked immunosorbent assay (ELISA)
d. Latex agglutination (LA)
e. Radioimmunoassay (RIA)

489. Inert particles are sensitized with either antigen or antibody. Which of the following tests is used extensively to detect microbial antigens rapidly (five minutes or less)?

a. Coagglutination (COA)
b. Counterimmunoelectrophoresis (CIE)
c. Enzyme-linked immunosorbent assay (ELISA)
d. Latex agglutination (LA)
e. Radioimmunoassay (RIA)

490. Its detection system is based on enzymatic activity. Which of the following tests is a heterogeneous immunoassay?

a. Coagglutination (COA)
b. Counterimmunoelectrophoresis (CIE)
c. Enzyme-linked immunosorbent assay (ELISA)
d. Latex agglutination (LA)
e. Radioimmunoassay (RIA)

Item 491–495

The diagram presents the various steps (labeled A–F) of the enzyme immunoassay.

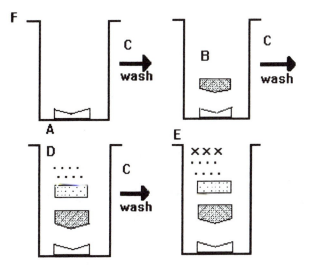

491. Failure of or improper methods for which step in the process will be the primary cause of high background color?

a. A
b. B
c. C
d. D
e. E
f. F

492. Where is unlabeled antibody attached if this enzyme immunoassay is intended for detection of antigen?

a. A
b. B
c. C
d. D
e. E
f. F

493. What is the location of the "solid phase"?

a. A
b. B
c. C
d. D
e. E
f. F

494. Addition of reagent at which step will cause color in the positive control well and reactive patient specimens?

a. A
b. B
c. C
d. D
e. E
f. F

495. What is the location of the patient specimen in the diagram?

a. A
b. B
c. C
d. D
e. E
f. F

496. An 18-year-old male patient with acute lymphocytic leukemia fails all standard chemotherapies. Cells from an HLA-nonidentical donor are used to perform a bone marrow transplant. Prior to transplantation, the patient is given broad-spectrum antibiotics and an immunosuppressive regimen. Within two to four weeks, lymphocyte and granulocyte numbers begin to rise, confirming bone marrow cell engraftment. However, one month later, the patient develops diarrhea, jaundice, and a severe maculopapular rash. Physical exam reveals hepotomegaly and splenomegaly. Which of the following is most likely occurring?

a. Acute rejection
b. Chronic rejection
c. Cyclosporine A toxicity
d. Graft-versus-host disease (GVHD)
e. Hyperacute rejection

497. A 27-year-old male patient (blood group O) arrives at the emergency room with a massive intestinal bleed (hematochezia). Within hours he has lost half of his blood volume, and you decide to transfuse. Due to human error, you transfuse blood, group AB, into him and within minutes he develops a fever, chills, dyspnea, and a dramatic drop in blood pressure. This reaction is most likely due to which of the following?

a. A cell-mediated response against AB antigens
b. IgG production by the recipient in response to AB antigens
c. Preformed anti-A and anti-B antibodies in the recipient
d. Preformed anti-A and anti-B antibodies of the blood donor
e. Preformed isohemagglutinins of the IgG isotype

Questions 498–500

498. During a clinic office visit, a 35-year-old male stockbroker shows signs of excessive nervousness and irritability and complains that the office is too hot. History and physical reveal the presence of a goiter and exophthalmia. Laboratory analysis of his blood reveals high antibody titers against the thyroid-stimulating hormone (TSH) receptor. Which of the following diseases does this patient have?

a. Goodpasture's syndrome
b. Grave's disease
c. Hashimoto's disease
d. Juvenile onset diabetes mellitus
e. Myasthenia gravis
f. Pernicious anemia
g. Rheumatoid arthritis
h. Systemic lupus erythematosus (SLE)

499. A 9-year-old female with a recent history of weight loss and vision problems arrives at the hospital. Soon after, it is determined that she has low blood glucose, and autoantibodies against beta cells are detected in her serum. Which of the following diseases does this patient have?

a. Goodpasture's syndrome
b. Grave's disease
c. Hashimoto's disease
d. Juvenile onset diabetes mellitus
e. Myasthenia gravis
f. Pernicious anemia
g. Rheumatoid arthritis
h. Systemic lupus erythematosus (SLE)

500. A 35-year-old woman with fever, weight loss, fatigue, and painful joints and muscles presents to her physician's office. The physician notes that she has marked photosensitivity and a rash on the cheeks and over the bridge of her nose. Laboratory tests reveal anemic conditions and the presence of anti-DNA antibodies. Which one of the following is the correct diagnosis for this patient?

a. Goodpasture's syndrome
b. Grave's disease
c. Hashimoto's disease
d. Juvenile onset diabetes mellitus
e. Myasthenia gravis
f. Pernicious anemia
g. Rheumatoid arthritis
h. Systemic lupus erythematosus (SLE)

Immunology

Answers

410–413. The answers are 410-h, 411-c, 412-c, 413-d. *(Parslow, pp 197–202, 380, 386–388. Levinson, pp 414–421.)* The diagrams in 1, 2, 3, and 4 represent Type I, II, III, and IV hypersensitivity, respectively. The table below describes these reactions in detail.

	HYPERSENSITIVITY REACTIONS	
Mediator	**Type**	**Reaction**
Antibody (IgE)	I (immediate, anaphylactic)	IgE antibody is induced by allergen and binds to mast cells and basophils. When exposed to the allergen again, the allergen cross-links the bound IgE, which induces degranulation and release of mediators, e.g., histamine.
Antibody (IgG)	II (cytotoxic)	Antigens on a cell surface combine with antibody; this leads to complement-mediated lysis, e.g., transfusion or Rh reactions, or autoimmune hemolytic anemia.
Antibody (IgG)	III (immune complex)	Antigen-antibody immune complexes are deposited in tissues, complement is activated, and polymorphonuclear cells are attracted to the site. They release lysosomal enzymes, causing tissue damage.
Cell	IV (delayed)	Helper T lymphocytes sensitized by an antigen release lymphokines upon second contact with the same antigen. The lymphokines induce inflammation and activate macrophages, which, in turn, release various mediators.

Reprinted, with permission, from Levinson W, Jawetz E. Medical Microbiology, 7e. New York: McGraw-Hill, 2002, 415.

414–415. The answers are 414-b, 415-a. *(Parslow, pp 117, 302–305. Levinson, pp 431, 432.)* Bruton's agammaglobulinemia is a congenital defect that becomes apparent at approximately six months of age, when maternal IgG is diminished. It occurs in males and is characterized by a defective btk gene, very small tonsils, low levels of all five classes of immunoglobulins, and no mature B cells. Thus, the child is unable to produce immunoglobulins and develops a series of bacterial infections characterized by recurrences and progression to more serious infections such as septicemia. The most common organisms responsible for infection are *H. influenzae* and *S. pneumoniae.* Cell-mediated immunity is not affected, and the child is able to respond normally to diseases that require this immune response for resolution. Treatment consists of pooled IgG.

Note: Immunodeficiency is characterized by unusual and recurrent infections:

- B cell (antibody) deficiency—bacterial infections
- T cell deficiency—viral, fungal, and protozoal infections
- Phagocytic cell deficiency—pyogenic infections (bacterial), skin infections, systemic bacterial opportunistic infections
- Complement deficiencies—pyogenic infections (bacterial)

416. The answer is d. *(Parslow, pp 3–5.)* The primary constituent cells of the immune system are bone-marrow-derived lymphocytes (B cells) and thymus-derived lymphocytes (T cells). Cytokines are polypeptides that modulate the function of immunoresponsive cells, and interleukins are cytokines that are produced by mononuclear cells. Platelets, derived from the myeloid pathway of hematopoiesis, appear not to be immunoresponsive and are involved in blood clotting.

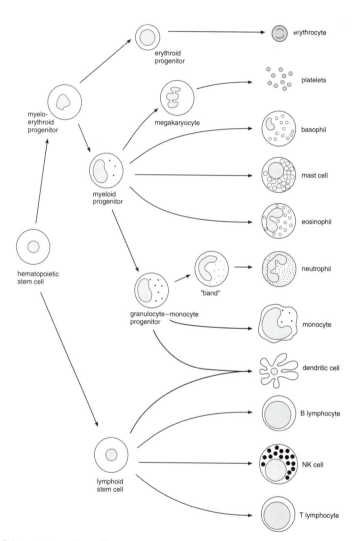

Schematic overview of hematopoiesis, emphasizing the erythroid, myeloid, and lymphoid pathways. This highly simplified depiction omits many recognized intermediate cell types in each pathway. All of the cells shown here develop to maturity in the bone marrow, except T lymphocytes, which develop from marrow-derived progenitors that migrate to the thymus. A common lymphoid stem cell serves as the progenitor of T and B lymphocytes and of natural killer (NK) cells. Dendritic cells arise from both the myeloid and lymphoid lineages. (*Reproduced, with permission, from Parslow TG et al.* Medical Immunology, *10e. New York: McGraw-Hill, 2001, 3.*)

417. The answer is b. (*Parslow, p 62. Levinson, pp 375–376, 382, 384–385.*) The great heterogeneity in the B cell response is characterized by a wide variety of antigenic stimuli. The end result of this remarkable process is a set of very specific surface receptors on B lymphocytes. However, it is the hypervariable regions in the variable domain of these B cells that provide the amino acid residues that confer specificity by synthesis of surface immunoglobulin receptors. T cells, on the other hand, do not secrete immunoglobulins.

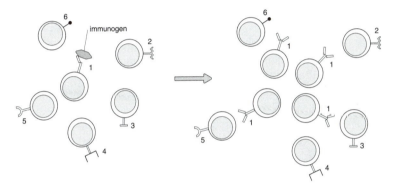

Clonal selection of lymphocytes by a specific immunogen. **Left:** The unimmunized lymphocyte population is composed of cells from many different clones, each with its own antigen specificity, indicated here by the distinctive shapes of the surface antigen receptors. **Right:** Contact with an immunogen leads to selective proliferation (positive selection) of any clone or clones that can recognize that specific immunogen. (*Reproduced, with permission, from Parslow TG et al. Medical Immunology, 10e. New York: McGraw-Hill, 2001, 62.*)

418. The answer is a. (*Parslow, pp 79–80, 700–703. Levinson, pp 82, 146, 429.*) Recurrent severe infection is an indication for clinical evaluation of immune status. Live vaccines, including BCG attenuated from M. *tuberculosis*, should not be used in the evaluation of a patient's immune competence because patients with severe immunodeficiencies may develop an overwhelming infection from the vaccine. For the same reason, oral (Sabin) polio vaccine is not advisable for use in such persons.

419. The answer is e. (*Parslow, p 625. Levinson, p 268.*) Measles-like virus has been isolated from the brain cells of patients with SSPE. The role of the host immune response in the causation of SSPE has been supported by several findings including the following: (1) progression of disease despite high levels of humoral antibody; (2) presence of a factor that blocks lymphocyte-mediated immunity to SSPE-measles virus in SSPE cerebrospinal fluid (CSF); (3) lysis of brain cells from SSPE patients by SSPE serum or CSF in the presence of complement (a similar mechanism could cause in vivo tissue injury). SSPE is particularly common in those who acquired measles before two years of age and is very rare after measles vaccination.

Higher-than-normal levels of serum antibodies (Ab) to measles virus and local synthesis of measles Ab in CSF, as evidenced by the oligoclonal IgG, imply a connection between the virus and multiple sclerosis (MS). However, the other studies have implicated the other viruses. Several studies of cell-mediated hypersensitivity to measles and other viruses in MS have been done, but the results have been conflicting. Definite conclusions regarding defects in cellular immunity in this disease cannot be reached until further research is completed.

420. The answer is b. (*Parslow, pp 84–85, 275. Levinson, pp 395, 397–398.*) In the question presented, the haplotypes of the father are 3,25 and 7,12 and the haplotypes of the mother are 1,3 and 8,9. (A haplotype is composed of one allele—antigen—from the one gene of a pair and one allele from the other gene.) Each child of this couple would have inherited one haplotype from each parent. Thus, possible offspring haplotypes are (1) 3,25; 1,3; (2) 3,25; 8,9; (3) 7,12; 1,3; and (4) 7,12; 8,9.

421. The answer is e. (*Parslow, pp 251–252.*) The graph presented in the question exhibits hemagglutinating antibody responses to primary and secondary immunization with any standard antigen. Curve B represents the early response to primary immunization, which is chiefly an IgM response. Rechallenge elicits an accelerated response that mainly involves IgG and occurs two to five days after reimmunization. IgM has a molecular weight of 900,000 and is a pentamer that the fetus can produce quite early in gestation. IgM (and IgG) have the ability to activate complement, appear along with sIgD as the B cell receptor on B lymphocytes, and like IgA require J chains to join the Fc chains of each monomer together.

422. The answer is e. *(Parslow, pp 215–217. Levinson, pp 404–405.)* The ascending limb A of the precipitin curve presented in the question represents the zone of antibody excess; in this zone, the supernatant solution would contain unreacted antibody. On the descending limb C, or the antigen-excess zone, the supernatant solution contains excess free antigen. In a monospecific system, B designates the region of maximum precipitation, and the supernatant solution is free to precipitate antibody and antigen. In a complex multispecific system, excess antigen or antibody molecules may be present at the point of maximum precipitate formation because the optimal quantity of each antigen may be different.

423. The answer is a. *(Parslow, pp 221–223. Levinson, pp 58, 406, 408.)* ELISA (enzyme-linked immunosorbent assay) methods can be used to detect either antigens or antibodies. If antigen is to be detected, then specific antibody is initially bound to the plate (see A in the diagram presented with the question). If antibody is to be detected, then antigen is bound to the solid phase. The bound antigen and antibody then "captures" the analyte to be detected. One of the major causes for high background in ELISA tests is the failure to wash off unbound antigen or antibody (see B in the diagram presented with the question). ELISA is routinely used to screen patient sera for different antibodies (including anti-HIV-1 antibodies). In this case, the well is initially coated with HIV-1 antigen and the patient sera is tested for anti-HIV-1 antibodies.

424. The answer is a. *(Parslow, pp 216, 218. Levinson, pp 405, 407.)* In the Ouchterlony agar-gel diffusion test, an antigen and a series of antibodies (or an antibody and a series of antigens) are allowed to diffuse toward each other. At the zone of optimal proportions of the reactants, a precipitin line occurs. Cross-reactions between antigens or antibodies tested can be detected by (1) a shortening of the major precipitin band contiguous to the cross-reacting substance, or (2) the identity of precipitin reaction between the two cross-dressing substances. The figures presented in the question illustrate both types of cross-reaction. In the first bleed pattern shown in the question, cross-reaction between antigen X and antigen A is recognizable only by a shortening of the precipitin band between the center well and X on the A well side (relative to the band going directly into the normal saline well). In the second bleed pattern, full cross-reaction of X and A is apparent. No other cross-reactions are seen.

425. The answer is a. (*Parslow, p 334. Levinson, pp 49, 378, 432, 434.*) The patient in this case has chronic granulomatous disease (CGD), an X-linked (65%) or autosomal recessive (35%) inherited disease. Patients with CGD are not able to generate a respiratory burst after granulocyte and monocyte stimulation. Thus, they are unable to kill microorganisms. Answers a, b, and c are all involved in the respiratory burst; however, the central enzyme is the NADPH oxidase (answer a). Without this enzyme, hydrogen peroxide (answer b), superoxide (answer c), and other microbial reactive oxygen species would not be generated.

426. The answer is b. (*Parslow, pp 113–114. Levinson, pp 221, 227–228, 279.*) Immunoglobulin gene rearrangement errors can contribute to the development of many types of leukemia and lymphoma. Some genetic alterations are characteristic of particular histologic entities: t(8;14) in Burkitt's lymphoma, t(14;18) in follicular lymphoma, t(11;14) in mantle cell lymphoma, and t(2;5) in anaplastic large cell lymphoma.

427. The answer is c. (*Parslow, pp 82–83. Levinson, p 395.*) The figure shown in the question is a schematic representation of the MHC Class I molecule, which has a CD8 binding site ($\alpha3$) and a peptide-binding site ($\alpha1$ and $\alpha2$). MHC Class I is active on all nucleated cells.

428. The answer is a. (*Parslow, pp 101–102. Levinson, pp 382, 384.*) The initial response to a new infection is with an IgM class antibody. IgM develops quickly and usually disappears within a few months. The secondary response is IgG and reflects the patient's immune status or, in the case of chickenpox, a vaccination given.

429–431. The answers are 429-e, 430-a, 431-a. (*Levinson, pp 286–294, 461.*) A male patient with the presentation as outlined in question 429 (fatigue, weight loss, and lymphadenopathy) must be tested for antibodies to HIV. While other antibody tests may be relevant after the primary diagnosis, they must be considered after HIV is ruled out. Certainly, infectious mononucleosis is a possibility, but its occurrence in this age group is not as frequent as HIV. Patients are tested first by an ELISA screening test. If this test is positive (X2), then a confirmatory western blot is performed. A western blot separates the immune response into antibody production for specific components of the virus, that is, envelope, gag, and so forth. The following table shows the various bands that could be seen on a widely used western blot and their identification by specific antigen source. There are at least three schemes for interpreting western blots. Assuming technical competence in the laboratory, one of the more common reasons for falsely positive ELISAs and western blots is an influenza vaccination within the past few months. A rare patient may have antibody to the cell line used to grow virus. Unlike Lyme disease, there is no reported cross-reactivity with Epstein-Barr virus (EBV) or HTLV. There appears to be no naturally occurring antibody to retroviruses.

Antigen	Source
gp 160	Env gene product
gp 120	Env fragment
gp 41	Transmembrane fragment
gp 31	
gp 51	Pol gene product
p 66	
p 24	Core protein (gag)

Abbreviations: gp, glycoprotein; p, protein; env, envelope; pol, polymerase.

432. The answer is d. *(Parslow, p 344. Levinson, p 433.)* Patients with complement deficiencies such as C5 through C9, which form the membrane attack complex (MAC), are predisposed to disseminated meningococcal disease. These patients may also be susceptible to gonococcal infection. There appears to be no disposition to AIDS or to fungal, parasitic, or pneumococcal infections.

433. The answer is d. *(Parslow, pp 23–24. Levinson, pp 47, 359, 379, 399, 428.)* The acute-phase response is a primitive, nonspecific defense reaction, mediated by the liver, that increases innate immunity and other protective functions in stressful times. It can be triggered by chronic autoimmune disorders such as rheumatoid arthritis and Crohn's disease. This response occurs when hepatocytes are exposed to IL-6 and IL-1 of TNF-α. LPS is a potent inducer of these cytokines. They are responsible for fever, somnolence, loss of appetite, and, if the response is prolonged, anemia and cachexia (wasting). A traditional assay known as the *erythrocyte sedimentation rate* (ESR) may be used as an indicator of an acute-phase response. The ESR involves measuring the rate at which the red blood cells fall through plasma, which increases as fibrinogen concentration rises. Currently, Crohn's disease may be treated with infusions of a drug known as Infliximab which is a mouse-human chimeric antibody against human TNF-α.

434. The answer is d. *(Parslow, p 703. Levinson, pp 50–51, 353, 355, 357, 359.)* Natural immunity is nonspecific. The natural immune functions described are not specific for a certain antigen. For example, certain proteins such as C-reactive protein (CRP) are acute-phase reactants. While elevated CRP is seen in infection, it is not disease-specific. Maternal transfer of antibody, however, is passive but still confers specific immunity. It is termed *acquired* immunity.

435. The answer is b. *(Parslow, pp 76–77. Levinson, pp 360–361.)* Haptens (incomplete antigens) are not themselves antigenic, but when coupled to a cell or carrier protein become antigenic and induce antibodies that can bind the hapten alone (in the absence of the carrier protein). They are small molecules that are generally less than 1000 Da. While haptens react with antibodies, they are not immunogenic because they do not activate T cells and cannot bind the major histocompatibility complex (MHC). Haptens are significant in disease; penicillin is a hapten and can cause severe life-threatening allergic reaction by destruction of erythrocytes. Catechols in the oils of poison ivy plants are haptens and cause a significant skin inflammatory response. Chloramphenicol is a hapten that can lead to the destruction of leukocytes and cause agranulocytosis. Sedormid is a hapten that can cause thrombocytopenia and purpura (bleeding) through the destruction of platelets.

436. The answer is d. *(Parslow, p 131. Ryan, pp 115–119.)* T cells do not synthesize antibody; that is the task of B cells. Recognition of certain epitopes, lymphokine production, and eradication of "foreign cells" are all functions of T cells. One of the best-recognized T cells is the CD4 cell. The importance of CD4 cells to the immune response is demonstrated by the effects of a specific inhibition of CD4 functions, that is, human immunodeficiency virus (HIV).

437. The answer is b. *(Parslow, pp 95–97, 101. Ryan, pp 124–127.)* The hinge region consists mostly of cysteine and proline residues, allowing for the formation of interchain disulphide bonds and flexibility, respectively. There appears to be considerable flexibility in the hinge region between the Fc and the two F(ab) portions of the molecule. This allows the molecule to assume either a T shape or a Y shape. The two arms of the antibody are identical and possess the same paratopes; hence, they will recognize identical epitopes. Each variable and constant heavy and light chains consist of the same amino acid sequences. IgG is the most abundant antibody in the serum. It migrates in the gamma globulin fraction during serum protein separation and composes 80% of the antibody concentration in the serum. Two enzymes, papain and pepsin, can digest an IgG antibody molecule by cleaving (hydrolysis) the antibody molecule on the N and C terminus sides, respectively, of the sulfhydryl bridge binding the heavy chains. Finally, antibodies protect the host by neutralization (preventing adherence), opsonizing (promoting phagocytosis), and activating complement (lysis).

Schematic model of an IgG1 (κ) human antibody molecule showing the basic four-chain structure and domains (V_H, C_H1, etc.). Sites of enzymatic cleavage by pepsin and papain are shown. (*Reproduced, with permission, from Parslow TG et al. Medical Immunology, 10e. New York: McGraw-Hill, 2001, 96.*)

438. The answer is d. (*Parslow, p 637. Levinson, p 287.*) HIV-2 disease is very rare in the United States. However, HIV-2 is present in Africa, the Far East, and some parts of the Caribbean. Many of the screening tests for HIV-1 will not detect antibodies to HIV-2. Either a separate HIV-2 antibody test or a combination HIV-1/2 is necessary. While HTLV disease is also seen in the same geographic areas, the symptoms displayed by this patient are more akin to HIV disease. While an HIV-1 RNA PCR is a useful test for monitoring the results of HIV therapy, it is not approved for diagnosis, nor will it detect HIV-2 nucleic acid.

439. The answer is c. (*Parslow, pp 143–144, 146. Levinson, pp 377–378.*) NK cells do not express a cell surface TCR/CD3 complex and are CD4–. About half of human NK cells are CD8+. Also, most NK cells express an Fc IgG receptor, known as CD16, and CD56, a neural cell adhesion molecule variant. NK cells are generally CD16+, CD56+, and CD3–, which contrasts them with T cells which are CD3+, CD16–, and CD56–.

440. The answer is e. (*Parslow, pp 175, 183–184. Levinson, pp 11, 400, 402. Ryan, p 49.*) C3a and C5a are potent mediators of inflammation; that is, they have anaphylatoxic activity. This activity is characterized by smooth-muscle contraction and the degranulation of mast cells and basophils leading to the release of histamine and other vasoactive substances, causing increased vascular (capillary) permeability. C5a is the most potent of these anaphylatoxins; however, it also serves another role as a potent chemotactic agent, attracting polymorphonucleated neutrophils and macrophages to the site of inflammation.

441. The answer is d. (*Jawetz, pp 350–351. Levinson, chapter 33. Parslow, pp 160–161.*) Alpha and beta interferons are proteins that can induce an antiviral state in uninfected cells via the production of secondary protein factors that inhibit viral protein synthesis by degrading only viral mRNA (not host mRNA). Also, they can increase the expression of MHC Class I proteins, which enable an infected cell to present viral antigens and facilitate killing by CTLs, and they can stimulate the production of gamma interferon. In addition, gamma interferon increases MHC Class II expression and antigen presentation in all cells and activates NK cells to kill virus-infected cells. Interferons have no direct effect on extracellular virus particles.

442. The answer is a. (*Parslow, p 721.*) Allograft rejection is primarily a T cell response to foreign tissue. The corticosteroids reduce inflammatory response and are generally administered by cytotoxic drugs, such as cyclosporine. Lymphoid irradiation is usually done so that the bone marrow is shielded. This removes lymphocytes from lymph nodes and spleen while allowing the patient to have the capacity to regenerate new T and B cells. Likewise, antilymphocyte globulin will destroy the recipient's lymphocytes, especially T cells. Destruction of donor B cells and T cells would not play a role in the immunosuppression of the graft recipient. In graft crises, monoclonal antibody to CD3 is sometimes given. This targets mature T lymphocytes for destruction.

443. The answer is c. (*Levinson, pp 377, 391.*) With repeated immunization, higher titers of all antibodies are observed, and, as priming is repeated, the immune response recruits B cells of progressively greater affinity. The affinity of antibody for a hapten-protein complex rises, cross-reactivity also rises, and the response becomes wider in specificity. As the number of antigenic sites detected per reacting particle increases, the avidity increases. In addition to shifts in the class of immunoglobulin synthesized in response to an antigen (IgM to IgG), shifts also may occur in the idiotype of antibody.

444. The answer is c. (*Levinson, pp 404–406.*) In precipitation reactions, both the antigen and the antibody are soluble. The antibody cross-links antigen molecules, creating an increasing lattice that eventually forms an insoluble precipitate. The antigen must be divalent, and the antigen/antibody proportion is critical in order for detectable precipitate to form. The prozone is the zone of antibody excess. The postzone is the zone of antigen excess. The zone of equivalence is the zone where the proportion of antibody and antigen is optimal for precipitate formation. Titer is the reciprocal of the highest dilution (ratio) of antibody (or antigen) at which there is still a detectable reaction.

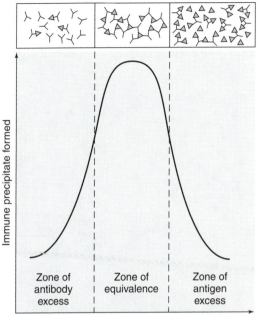

Increasing antigen concentration

Modified and reproduced, with permission, from Stites D, Terr A, Parslow T (eds.) Basic and Clinical Immunology, 9e. Originally published by Appleton & Lange. Copyright © 1997 by The McGraw-Hill Companies.)

445. The answer is b. *(Parslow, pp 207–209. Levinson, 384–387.)* Each secretory IgA molecule has a molecular weight of 400,000 and consists of two H2L2 units and one molecule each of J chain and secretory component. Some IgA exists in serum as a monomer H2L2 with a molecular weight of 160,000. Some bacteria, such as *Neisseria,* can destroy IgA-1 by producing protease. It is the major immunoglobulin in milk, saliva, tears, mucus, sweat, gastric fluid, and colostrum. IgA does not fix complement, so one would anticipate that a complement fixation test would not be useful for IgA antibody.

446. The answer is d. *(Parslow, pp 380–383.)* Both IgG and IgM activate complement by the classic pathway, while IgA activates it by the alternative pathway. IgA, IgD, and IgE cannot activate complement. Complement is a system of several proteins that is activated by either an immune or a non-immune pathway. Both of these pathways result in the production of many biologically active components that cause cell lysis and death.

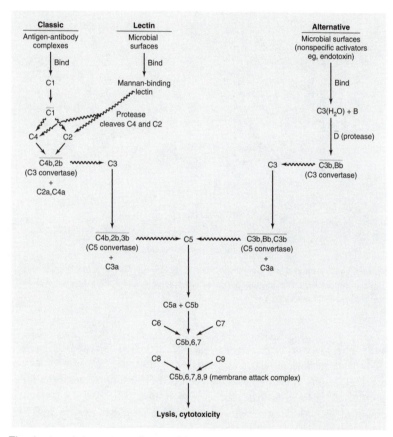

The classic and alternative pathways of the complement system. ⤳ indicates that proteolytic cleavage of the molecule at the tip of the arrow has occurred; a line over a complex indicates that it is enzymatically active. Note that the nomenclature of the cleavage products of C2 is undecided. Some call the large fragment C2a and others call it C2b. The C3 convertase is depicted here as C4b,2b. Note that proteases associated with the mannose-binding lectin cleave C4 as well as C2. (Reprinted, with permission, from Levinson W, Jawetz E. Medical Microbiology and Immunology, 7e. New York: McGraw-Hill, 2002, 401.)

447–451. The answers are 447-d, 448-c, 449-e, 450-b, 451-a.
(Parslow, pp 95–114. Levinson, pp 382–392.) IgG antibody provides an "immune history." That is, IgG antibody persists in most people and indicates the antigens to which they have been exposed. IgG is not formed early in infection but is a secondary response arising weeks to months after antigenic challenge. IgG also has a built-in memory. Even people with very low levels of specific IgG will respond to an antigen challenge with an IgG response.

IgM antibody, in contrast, arises early in infection and then disappears within a couple of months. IgM is intravascular and does not cross the placental barrier. For this reason, infants with specific IgG responses to disease must be tested for IgM to determine whether their immune systems have produced antibody or whether the test was positive because of passively transferred IgG.

IgA antibody is involved in local immunity at the level of the mucous membrane. IgA antibody also arises early in disease. IgA antibody is short-lived and will disappear similarly to IgM.

IgE antibody is characteristically seen in parasitic infections, particularly worm (helminth) infections because of the attraction of eosinophils to the site of the infestation. Certain allergies are due to excessive production of IgE.

IgD antibody consists of two light chains and two heavy chains. Its role is not known, but it can be found on the surface of lymphocytes, where it may act as a surface receptor.

IgG is susceptible to proteolytic enzymes, which may explain why it is present in such low levels in serum.

452–456. The answers are 452-a, 453-b, 454-e, 455-c, 456-d.
(Parslow, p 692.) B. burgdorferi, the causative agent of Lyme disease, elicits an acute antibody response. IgM appears within days to a few weeks following tick bite, and IgG appears a few weeks later. IgG persists; IgM does not. Cross-reactions occur with other treponemes.

Fifth disease is a viral exanthem commonly seen in children 8 to 12 years old. Children are ill for a few days but recover without incident. Unfortunately, if a pregnant female acquires the disease in the first trimester of pregnancy, the fetus is at risk. The causative agent is thought to be a Parvovirus (Parvovirus B19).

Adults with no titer to varicella (VZV) are at risk for acquisition of chickenpox. If they are health care workers, there is additional risk in transmitting VZV to immunodeficient children. Antibodies to VZV are readily detected by both enzyme immunoassay (EIA) and fluorescent antibody (FA) techniques.

Delta agent is a recently discovered antigen associated with HBsAg. Its presence usually correlates with HBsAg chronic carriers who have chronic active hepatitis. EIA and radioimmunoassay (RIA) tests are available to detect antibodies to delta agent.

SSPE is thought to be caused by a measles-related virus present in the central nervous system. Most SSPE patients show elevated measles virus antibodies in serum and CSF. In patients with multiple sclerosis (MS), lower CSF antibody titers have been observed, suggesting a possible etiologic role for measles virus in MS.

457–461. The answers are 457-d, 458-c, 459-d, 460-b, 461-d. (*Levinson, pp 431–436.*) Immunodeficiency disorders can be categorized according to whether the defect primarily involves humoral immunity (bone marrow–derived, or B lymphocytes) or cellular immunity (thymus-derived, or T lymphocytes) or both. Swiss-type hypogammaglobulinemia, ataxia-telangiectasia, the Wiskott-Aldrich syndrome, and severe combined immunodeficiency disorders all involve defective B cell and T cell function. Infantile X-linked agammaglobulinemia is caused chiefly by deficient B cell activity, whereas thymic hypoplasia is mainly a T cell immunodeficiency disorder.

462–465. The answers are 462-a, 463-b, 464-c, 465-d. (*Levinson, p 396.*) Transplantation from one region of a person to another region of that same person is an *autograft* and has the best chance of succeeding. When a transplant is done between monozygotic twins, it is an *isograft* and has a complete MHC compatibility and a good chance of success. *Allografts* are between members of the same species, and *xenografts* are between members of different species. Both of these transplants have a high rate of rejection unless immunosuppression accompanies the transplant.

466–468. The answers are 466-d, 467-c, 468-b. (*Levinson, pp 386–388.*) Isotypes are determined by antigens of the immunoglobulin classes found in all individuals of one species. In addition to heavy-chain isotypes of IgA, IgD, IgE, IgG, and IgM, two light-chain isotypes exist for κ and λ chains.

Allotypes are differentiated by antigenic determinants that vary among individuals within a species and are recognized by cross-immunization of individuals in a species. Allotypes include the Gm marker of IgG and the Inv marker of light chains.

Idiotypes are antigenic determinants that appear only on the F(ab) fragments of antibodies and appear to be localized at the ligand-binding site; thus, anti-idiotype antisera may block reactions with the appropriate hapten. The carbohydrate side chains of immunoglobulins are relatively nonimmunogenic. New determinants may be exposed after papain cleavage of immunoglobulins, but these determinants are not included in the classification of the native molecule.

469. The answer is e. *(Parslow, pp 376–379.)* This patient has a classic case of hereditary angioedema. This disease is characterized by a deficiency of complement control proteins such as C1 esterase inhibitor, leading to overactive complement. Uncontrolled generation of vasoactive peptides causes increased blood vessel permeability, causing hereditary angioedema. Edema, especially of the larynx, obstructs the airways. Abdominal pain may indicate that the patient has angioedema of the gut.

470. The answer is d. *(Parslow, pp 569–571. Harrison's, pp 252, 1632.)* The best-characterized human tumor-associated antigens are the oncofetal antigens. Carcinoembryonic antigen (CEA) is a glycoprotein and member of the immunoglobulin gene superfamily and is elevated in colorectal cancer. α-fetoprotein (AFP) is analogous to albumin and elevated in hepatocellular carcinoma. Prostate-specific antigen (PSA) is elevated in prostatic cancer. CEA, AFP, and PSA are all glycoproteins. Melena refers to altered (black) blood per rectum, indicative of an upper gastrointestinal bleed.

471–472. The answers are 471-b, 472-e. *(Parslow, pp 636, 638–642.)* HIV infection affects mainly the immune system and the brain. The main immunologic feature of HIV infection is progressive depletion of the CD4 subset of T lymphocytes (T helper cells), causing a reversal in the normal CD4:CD8 ratio, leading to immunodeficiency. Currently, ELISA is the basic screening test to detect anti-HIV antibodies. Repeated reactive ELISA tests should be confirmed using either western blot or immunofluorescence. The western blot detects specific antibodies against the various HIV proteins (antigens).

473. The answer is b. *(Levinson, pp 410–413. Parslow, pp 251, 252, 257.)* Anti-Rh antibodies (IgG are reactive at 37°C) are the leading cause of hemolytic disease of the newborn (HDN). Currently, Rh immunization can be suppressed in antepartum or postpartem Rh– women if high-titer anti-Rh immunoglobulin (RhIg) is administered within 72 hours after the potentially sensitizing dose of Rh+ cells (i.e., the birth of the child).

474–475. The answers are 474-g, 475-c. *(Parslow, pp 320–321.)* Immune deficiency disorders occur as a result of impaired function in one or more of the major immune system components such as B lymphocytes, T lymphocytes, B and T lymphocytes, phagocytic cells, and complement. Unusual and recurrent infections are the hallmark of immunodeficiency. SCID occurs as a result of an early defect in stem cell differentiation and may be caused as a result of defective IL-2 receptors, adenosine deaminase deficiency, or failure to make MHC Class II antigens. This condition is characterized by B and T cell deficiency and presents with recurrent infections. The other disorders listed do not have both B and T cell deficiency with an absence of a thymus gland. Definitive treatment of SCID consists of stem cell transplantation, with the ideal donor being a sibling with identical human leukocyte antigens (HLA).

476. The answer is b. *(Parslow, pp 575–576, 699–700, 703–706.)* There are three forms of immunity: active, passive, and adoptive. Active immunity involves an individual making his or her own antibodies either naturally, by infection, or artificially, by immunizations. Passive immunity refers to the transfer of preformed antibodies from one individual to another either naturally (transplacental or enteromammary antibodies from mother to fetus) or artificially through gamma globulin injections such as antitoxins, anti-Rh, and antivenoms (black widow spider bites, etc.). Finally, adoptive immunity refers to the transfer of lymphoid cells from an actively immunized donor and does not involve antibody transfer.

477. The answer is e. *(Harrison's, pp 1845–1847.)* Patients with T cell defects are generally susceptible to viral, fungal, and protozoan infections. This can be especially visible in patients with primary immunodeficiency diseases such as SCID. For further explanation of immunodeficiencies, please refer to the answer explanations for questions 413–414 and 473–474.

478–479. The answers are 478-c, 479-b. *(Parslow, p 217. Levinson, p 408. Ryan, p 245.)* The complement fixation (CF) test is a two-stage test. The first stage involves the union of antigen with its specific antibody, followed by the fixation of complement to the antigen-antibody structure. In order to determine whether complement has been "fixed," an indicator system must be employed to determine the presence of free complement. Free complement binds to the complexes formed when red blood cells (RBCs) are mixed with anti-RBC antibody; this binding causes lysis of the cells. Complement that has been fixed before addition of RBCs and anti-RBC antibody cannot cause lysis.

480. The answer is b. *(Parslow, pp 201–202, 370–372.)* This is an example of a type I hypersensitivity reaction. Type I hypersensitivity is also referred to as anaphylaxis or immediate-type hypersensitivity. Major components include IgE, mast cells/basophils, and pharmacologically active mediators. Exposure to antigen causes IgE production, followed by sensitization of mast cells and basophils. Subsequent encounter with the same allergen (antigen) leads to chemical mediator release (histamine, etc.) and also leads to clinical symptoms associated with asthma, allergic rhinitis, and so on. This reaction can occur within minutes and can be extremely severe and life-threatening.

481–485. The answers are 481-c, 482-a, 483-b, 484-e, 485-d. *(Parslow, pp 628–630. Levinson, pp 257–266. Ryan, pp 541–553.)* The following table presents the patterns of hepatitis B virus serologic markers observed in various stages of infection with HBV. The diagnosis of HBV infection is usually based on three tests: hepatitis B surface antigen, antibodies to surface antigen, and antibodies to core antigen. Tests are available, however, for e antigen and antibodies to e antigen. A variety of testing methods are available and include enzyme immunoassay, radioimmunoassay, hemagglutination, latex agglutination, and immune adherence. The delta agent has recently been described. The delta agent exacerbates infection with HBV, apparently in a synergistic manner. Commercial tests are now available for the delta agent.

	Serologic Markers					
Interpretation	HBsAg	Anti-HBeAg	IgM Anti-HBc	Total Anti-HBc	Anti-HBe	HBs
Acute infection						
Incubation period	+*	+*	–	–	–	–
Acute phase	+	+	+	+	–	–
Early convalescent phase	+	–	+	+	+	–
Convalescent phase	–	–	+	+	+	–
Late convalescent phase	–	–	–†	+	+	+
Long past infection	–	–	–	+‡	+ or –	+‡
Chronic infection						
Chronic active hepatitis	+§	+ or –	+ or –	+§	+ or –	–§
Chronic persistent hepatitis	+¶	+ or –	+ or –	+	+ or –	–
Chronic HBV carrier state	+¶	+ or –	+ or –	+	+ or –	–
HBsAg immunization	-	-	-	-	-	+

*HBsAg and HBeAg are occasionally undetectable in acute HBV infection.
†IgM anti-HBc may persist for over a year after acute infection when very sensitive assays are employed.
‡Total anti-HBc and anti-HBs may be detected together or separately long after acute infection.
§HBsAG-negative chronic active hepatitis may occur where total anti-HBc and anti-HBs may be detected together, separately, or not at all.
¶HBsAg-negative chronic persistent hepatitis and chronic HBV carriers have been observed.

486–490. The answers are 486-b, 487-a, 488-e, 489-d, 490-c.
(*Parslow, pp 219–227. Levinson, pp 404–413. Ryan, pp 243–249.*) Of the many methods available for antigen and antibody detection, LA, ELISA, RIA, CIE, and COA are the most widely used. Latex agglutination (LA) employs latex polystyrene particles sensitized by either antibody or antigen. LA is more sensitive than CIE and COA but slightly less sensitive than either RIA or EIA. LA has been used to detect *H. influenzae, Neisseria meningitidis,* and *S. pneumoniae* antigens in cerebrospinal fluid. LA has also been used for detection of cryptococcal antigen. Most recently, LA has been widely used for rapid detection of group A streptococcal antigen directly from the pharynx. The test is rapid (five minutes), sensitive (approximately 90%), and specific (99%).

Coagglutination (COA), also an agglutination test, is slightly less sensitive than LA but is less susceptible to changes in environment (e.g., temperature). Most strains of coagulase-positive staphylococci have protein A in their cell wall. Protein A binds the Fc fragment of microbial antigens in body fluids. COA has also been used to rapidly type or group bacterial isolates.

Enzyme immunoassays (EIAs) can be either homogeneous (EMIT) or heterogeneous (ELISA). EMIT has been used primarily for assays of low-molecular-weight drugs. Its primary use in microbiology has been for assays of aminoglycoside antibiotics. EIAs vary as to the solid support used. A variety of supports can be used, such as polystyrene microdilution plates, paddles, plastic beads, and tubes. The number of layers in the antibody-antigen sandwich varies; usually as additional layers are added, detection sensitivity is increased. The two most common enzymes are horseradish peroxidase (HRP) and alkaline phosphatase (AP). β-galactosidase has also been employed. Orthophenylene diamine is the most common substrate for HRP and p-nitrophenyl phosphate for AP. Because EIAs are usually read in the visible color range, the tests can be read qualitatively by eye or quantitatively by machine.

Counterimmunoelectrophoresis (CIE) was originally used for "Australia antigen" (HBsAg) but was soon replaced by RIA. For a decade, CIE was used to detect antigens in body fluids. CIE is not an easy technique. Its success depends on the control of many variables, including solid support, voltage, current, buffer, affinity and avidity of antibodies, charge on the antigen, and time of electrophoresing.

Radioimmunoassay involves the radiolabeling of either antibody or antigen (Ag) using ^{131}Iodine (^{131}I) or ^{125}I (radioisotopes). It measures very small quantities and can be used to detect hormones, carcinoembryonic antigen (CEA), hepatitis B Ag, steroids, prostaglandins, and morphine-related drugs in patient sera.

491–495. The answers are 491-c, 492-a, 493-f, 494-e, 495-b. *(Parslow, pp 221–224. Levinson, pp 406, 408. Ryan, pp 245–247.)* The enzyme immunoassay (EIA, ELISA) has become a common method for the detection of either antibody or antigen in a patient specimen. The technique is based on building a "sandwich." For example, the following sandwich is made on what is called the *solid phase*. The solid phase is usually a plastic microtiter plate but can be a plastic paddle or even a nitrocellulose membrane. First, whole *Toxoplasma* organisms or purified antigenic components of *Toxoplasma* are added to the plate and the plate is washed off Failure of one or more of the washing steps or inadequate washing usually causes high background color in the developed plate.

The *Toxoplasma* antigen-antibody complex must be detected by the addition of a second antibody to which is linked an enzyme such as horseradish peroxidase or alkaline phosphatase. The nature of this second antibody is dependent on whether one wishes to measure IgG or IgM. If the test is for IgG, then the second antibody is anti–human IgG conjugated to an enzyme. Following another wash cycle, the enzyme substrate is added to the plate and color develops in those wells where the sandwich is complete. If the patient's serum does not contain specific antibody, then the sandwich is not completed and there is no development of color. If the EIA is for detection of antigen, then the layers of the sandwich are as follows:

Specific antibody
Patient specimen (contain antigen)
Enzyme-labeled antibody specific for the antigen
Enzyme substrates

There are many variations of the test using a variety of antibodies, indicators such as fluorescence, and magnetic beads as solid phases. EIA is more sensitive than agglutination methods or complement fixation and slightly less sensitive than radioimmunoassay.

496. The answer is d. (*Parslow, pp 326–327, 739.*) GVHD occurs due to attack by the graft against the recipient. There are three requirements for GVHD rejection: (1) histocompatibility differences between the graft (donor) and host (recipient), (2) immunocompetent graft cells, and (3) immunodeficient host cell. Immunocompetent graft cells may be "passenger" lymphocytes or major cells transplanted and must be present in the graft. Prevention of GVHD is essential, as there is no adequate treatment once it is established.

497. The answer is c. (*Parslow, pp 254–255. Levinson, pp 410–413.*) All blood for transfusion should be carefully matched to avoid transfusion reaction. As shown in the tables below, persons with group O blood have no A or B antigens on their erythrocytes and are thus considered to be universal donors. In contrast, persons with group AB blood have neither A nor B antibody and thus are universal recipients.

ABO BLOOD GROUPS		
Group	**Antigen on Red Cell**	**Antibody in Plasma**
A	A	Anti-B
B	B	Anti-A
AB	A and B	No anti-A or anti-B
O	No A or B	Anti-A and anti-B

COMPATIBILITY OF BLOOD TRANSFUSIONS BETWEEN ABO BLOOD GROUPS*				
	Recipient			
Donor	**O**	**A**	**B**	**AB**
O	Yes	Yes	Yes	Yes
A (AA or AO)	No	Yes	No	Yes
B (BB or BO)	No	No	Yes	Yes
AB	No	No	No	Yes

*"Yes" indicates that a blood transfusion from a donor with that blood group to a recipient with that blood group is compatible, i.e., that no hemolysis will occur. "No" indicates that the transfusion is incompatible and that hemolysis of the donor's cells will occur.
Reprinted, with permission, from Levinson W, Jawetz E. Medical Microbiology and Immunology, 7e. New York: McGraw-Hill, 2002, 412.

498–500. The answers are 498-b, 499-d, 500-h. *(Parslow, pp 128–129, 401–405, 426–430. Levinson, pp 423–428. Harrison's, pp 1922–1925.)* Loss of tolerance by the immune system to certain self-components can lead to the formation of antibodies, causing tissue and organ damage. Such diseases are referred to as *autoimmune diseases.* There are a host of autoimmune diseases characterized by the autoantibodies. The presence of a "butterfly" rash is a classic cutaneous sign of SLE and is characterized by a rash over the bridge of the nose and on the cheeks.

Bibliography

Bhushan V, et al: *First Aid for the USMLE Step I,* New York, McGraw-Hill, 2002.

Braunwal E, et al (ed): *Harrison's Principles of Internal Medicine,* 15/e, New York, McGraw-Hill, 2001.

Brooks GF, et al (ed): Jawetz's *Medical Microbiology,* 22/e, New York, McGraw-Hill, 2001.

Levinson W, Jawetz E: *Medical Microbiology and Immunology,* 7/e, New York, McGraw-Hill, 2002.

Murray PR, et al (ed): *Manual of Clinical Microbiology,* 8/e, Washington, DC, ASM Press, 2003.

Murray PR, et al: *Medical Microbiology,* 4/e, St. Louis, Mosby, 2002.

Parslow TG, et al: *Medical Immunology,* 10/e, New York, McGraw-Hill, 2001.

Ryan KJ, et al (ed): *Sherris Medical Microbiology,* 4/e, New York, McGraw-Hill, 2001.

Index

A

Absidia, 10, 208
Acanthamoeba, 215, 234
Actinomyces species, 2
   A. israelii, 114, 129, 136, 151, 164, 168
   A. odontolyticus, 151
   A. viscosus, 137, 151, 168
Acute hemolytic anemia, 61, 92
Adenoviruses, 3, 57, 66, 71, 88, 92, 96, 99
   gastroenteritis cause, 102, 103
   specimen collection for detection, 74, 101
AIDS (acquired immunodeficiency syndrome)
   M. avium, 125, 161
   opportunistic infections, 211
   tests for, 49, 79
   therapy for, 50, 80
Allografts, 259, 265, 289–290, 294
Allotypes, 265, 295
Alphaviruses, 58, 88–89
Amebas, 11, 227, 240
Anemia, acute hemolytic, 61, 92
Anthrax, 31, 46
Antibiotics
   E. coli growth curves with, 26–27, 43
   focus of, 21, 40
   mechanisms of, 31–32, 46–47
   quinolones, 110, 146
   uses of, 129–130, 164–165
Antibodies, 12, 250, 283
   following vaccinations, 249, 282–283
Antimicrobial agents, 2, 9
Arboviruses, 51, 81
Ascaris, 12, 229, 242
Aspergillus species, 193, 196, 206, 208
   A. fumigatus, 10, 189, 194, 203, 207, 208
Astrovirus, 75, 102, 103
Autoantibodies, 14
Autografts, 264, 294
Autoimmune diseases, 276–277, 301

B

Babesia, 213, 232, 233, 244
Bacillus species
   B. anthracis, 6, 35, 47–48
   B. cereus, 6, 7, 122, 158
Bacteria, 5–8
  aggregates, 1
  control of, 2

Bacteria (*Cont.*):
  growth curves of, 2, 20–21, 25–26, 39, 43
  growth of, 28, 44
  media to isolate, 133–134, 166–167
  normal, 135, 167–168
  pathogenesis, 2
  shapes of, 1
  structures of, 1, 34–35, 47–48
  transfer of, 1, 27–28, 43–44
  transport, 2, 15, 36
Bacterial lipopolysaccharide (LPS), 35, 47–48
Bacteroides species, 2
   B. fragilis, 111, 135, 146–147, 168
   B. melaninogenicus, 147
Bartonella species, 8
   B. henselae, 123, 159–160, 180, 187
Basidiobolus, 208, 211
B cells, 13, 247, 281
Blastomyces dermatitidis, 10, 199, 210
Blood transfusions, 275, 300–301
Bordetella species, 140, 171
   B. bronchiseptica, 133, 166
   B. pertussis, 7, 137, 143, 169
Borrelia species, 7
   B. burgdorferi, 153, 227, 240–241, 262, 293
   B. recurrentis, 153
Botulism, 6, 118, 134, 154, 167
Bovine spongiform encephalopathy, 44–45, 59, 90
Branhamella, 127, 163–164
Brucella species, 7, 116, 139, 152, 170
   B. abortus, 132, 166
Bruton's agammaglobulinemia, 13, 246–247, 279
Bubonic plague, 30, 46, 123, 152, 159
Burkitt's lymphoma, 72, 100, 253, 284

C

Calicivirus, 102, 103
Campylobacter jejuni, 8, 118, 130, 155, 165
Candida species, 9, 200, 210
   C. albicans, 10, 193, 195, 200, 203, 205–206, 208, 211
Capnocytophaga, 128, 164
Carcinoembryonic antigen (CEA), 266, 295
Catalase catalyzes, 2, 9
Cat-scratch disease (CSD), 123, 159–160, 180, 187

Chickenpox, 4, 70, 83, 99, 262, 293–294
Chlamydia species, 8, 173, 178, 182, 186
   C. pneumoniae, 8, 140, 171, 178, 186
   C. psittaci, 8, 174, 175, 182, 183–184, 186
   C. trachomatis, 8, 174, 175, 176, 177, 180,
     183–184, 185–186, 188
   development cycle of, 175, 184
Chloramphenicol, 26, 43
Cholera, 117, 130–131, 154, 165–166
Clonorchis sinensis, 11, 222, 223, 236–237
Clostridium species, 2, 6, 119
   C. botulinum, 6, 118, 134, 154, 167
   C. difficile, 6, 113, 149–150, 165
   C. perfringens, 6, 122, 158
   C. tetani, 6, 126, 163
Coccidioides immitis, 10, 194, 195, 198, 201,
   206–207, 209, 211–212
Colorado tick fever, 90–91
Complement fixation antibody measurements,
   269, 297
Complement pathways, 260, 291–292
Complement system, 258, 289
Condyloma acuminatum, 64, 93
Conidiobolus, 211
Coronaviruses, 4, 52, 82
Corynebacterium diphtheria, 6, 120, 137, 156,
   168–169
Coxiella burnetii, 8, 164, 173, 181, 182, 183,
   187
Coxsackievirus, 60, 90–91, 95
Coxsackievirus A, 4, 83
Creutzfeldt-Jakob disease, 44, 56, 87, 90
Crohn's disease, 256, 285–286
Croup, 64, 93
Cryptococcus neoformans, 10, 189, 191, 203,
   204
Cryptosporidium, 11, 214, 233
Cyclospora, 122, 159, 214, 233
Cytokines, 13
Cytomegalovirus (CMV), 4, 61, 65, 68, 71,
   73, 92, 94, 98, 99–101

D
Delta agent, 52, 82, 262, 294
Dengue fever, 4, 67, 91, 97
Dermatophytes, 9–10, 192, 199–200, 205,
   210
DiGeorge's syndrome, 13–14, 264, 294
Diphtheria, 6, 7, 120, 137, 156, 168–169
Diphyllobothrium latum, 11, 225, 238–239
Dipicolinic acid, 19, 39

DNA, 25, 42
DNA viruses, 3, 3–4, 61, 91

E
Eastern equine encephalitis (EEE), 4, 56,
   86–87
Echinococcus species, 126, 162
   E. granulosus, 11, 224, 238
Echoviruses, 4, 53, 82, 95
Ehrlichia species, 8, 177, 185
   E. chaffeenis, 180, 185, 187
   E. ewingii, 184
   E. phagocytophilia, 184
ELISA (*see* Enzyme-linked immunosorbent
   assay [ELISA] test)
Endotoxins, 2, 7
Entamoeba histolytica, 11, 229, 240, 242
Enterococcus, 119, 128, 155, 164
Enterovirus, 53, 65, 73, 83, 95–96, 101
Enzyme-linked immunosorbent assay (ELISA)
   test, 13, 51, 81, 251, 255–256, 272,
   273–274, 283, 285, 299–300
Epidermophyton, 9, 192, 198, 199, 205, 209,
   210
Epstein-Barr virus, 4, 51, 58, 66, 67, 72, 81,
   89, 91, 96–97, 100–101
Escherichia coli, 6, 7, 16, 36
   enterotoxigenic *E. coli*, 123, 159
   growth curves, 20–21, 26–27, 39, 43
   growth of, 28, 44
   O157/H7, 122, 138, 159, 169
   porins, 22, 40
   spheroplasts, 24, 42
Eumycotic mycetoma, 191, 204
Exotoxins, 2, 7

F
Fifth disease, 262, 293
Flaviviruses, 4
Flukes, 11, 228, 231, 241, 244
Francisella tularenis, 7, 138, 152, 169
Fungal infections
   granuloma formation, 192, 205
   opportunistic infections, 10, 195–196,
     207–208
   thick walled spores, 190, 203
Fungi, 9–10, 198–199, 209–210

G
Gardnerella vaginalis, 7, 108, 142
Gastroenteritis, 74–75, 102, 103

Genes
  cloning, 25, 42
  mutations, 30, 45
German measles virus, 4, 56, 87
Giardia species, 217, 230, 232, 234, 243, 244
  G. lamblia, 11, 162, 218, 219, 229, 234, 235, 242
Graft-versus-host disease, 275, 300
Gram-negative bacilli, 6
Gram-negative bacteria, 1, 29, 44, 47–48
Gram-negative cocci, 6
Gram-negative diplococci, 111, 147
Gram-negative rods, 6, 132–133, 143, 166
Gram-positive bacilli, 6
Gram-positive bacteria, 1, 47–48
Gram-positive cocci, 5
Gram stains, 1, 21–22, 40
Grave's disease, 276, 301
Group B streptococcal (GBS) disease, 115–116, 151–152

H
Haemophilus species
  H. ducreyi, 7
  H. influenzae, 6, 107, 118, 142, 143, 155, 165
Hantavirus, 60, 91
Haplotypes, 248, 282
Haptens, 257, 286
Helicobacter pylori, 6, 8, 107, 124, 141, 160
Hematopoiesis, 247, 280
Hepatitis viruses
  diagnosis of, 270–271, 297–298
  hepatitis A (HAV), 3, 69, 74, 75, 99, 102
  hepatitis B (HBV), 3, 55, 57, 67–68, 70, 76, 85–86, 88, 91, 97–98, 102
  hepatitis C (HCV), 3, 67, 75, 91, 97, 102
  hepatitis D (HDV), 3, 55, 76, 85, 102
  hepatitis E (HEV), 3, 55, 60, 76, 84–85, 90, 102
Hereditary angioedema, 266, 295
Herpesvirus simplex virus, 3, 49, 58, 80, 89
  HSV-1, 3, 77, 80, 104
  HSV-2, 3, 80
  HSV meningitis, 53, 83
  specimen collection for detection, 101
  tests for, 17–18, 37–38
  treatment for, 70, 99

Histoplasma capsulatum, 10, 194, 202, 206, 212
HIV (human immunodeficiency virus)
  infectious disease risks, 50, 80–81
  risk of acquiring, 59, 89–90
  screening tests for, 51, 81, 255–256, 258, 267, 284–285, 288, 295
  structures of, 49, 79
  viral loads, 50, 80
Human granulocytic ehrlichiosis (HGE), 176, 177, 184, 185
Human monocytic ehrlichiosis (HME), 174, 177, 183, 195
Human papillomavirus (HPV), 54, 61, 64, 71, 73, 76, 84, 91, 92, 93, 99, 101, 104
Hypersensitivity reactions, 245–246, 270, 278, 297
  types of, 14

I
Idiotypes, 266, 295
Immune responses, 256, 286
  types of, 12, 14, 268, 296
Immunizations (*see* Vaccinations)
Immunodeficiency disorders, 13–14, 263–264, 268, 294, 296
  (*See also* AIDS [acquired immunodeficiency syndrome]; HIV [human immunodeficiency virus])
Immunoglobulins, 12–13, 257, 287
  IgA, 12, 260, 261, 291, 293
  IgD, 12, 13, 261, 293
  IgE, 12, 13, 261, 293
  IgG, 12, 254, 262, 284, 288, 293
  IgM, 12, 13, 261, 262, 293
Immunologic tests, 271–272, 298–299
  (*See also* Enzyme-linked immunosorbent assay [ELISA] test)
Influenza, 5
  diagnosis of, 66, 96, 140, 170
  H. influenzae, 6, 107, 118, 142, 143, 155, 165
  interferon and, 52, 82
  vaccinations for, 70, 98
Inhalation anthrax, 31, 46
Interferon, 52, 65, 82, 95, 259, 289
Isografts, 264, 294
Isotypes, 265, 294

J
JC virus, 104

K

Koch's postulates, 1, 28, 44
Kuru, 56, 87

L

Lactobacillus, 135, 168
Latex agglutination (LA) test, 121, 157, 272, 298
Legionella pneumophila, 7, 113, 129, 140, 143, 148–149, 165, 170–171
Leptospirosis, 134, 153, 167
Lice, 225, 239
Listeria monocytogenes, 6, 111, 126, 148, 163
Löwenstein-Jensen medium, 134, 166–167
Lyme disease, 22, 41, 124, 129, 160–161, 165, 227, 240–241, 262, 293
Lymphocytes, 281
Lymphogranuloma venereum (LGV), 175, 177, 180, 183, 186, 188

M

Mad cow disease, 44–45, 59, 90
Major histocompatability complex (MHC), 13, 254, 284
Malassezia furfur, 9, 200, 210
Measles virus, 4, 54, 84, 93
    complement fixation antibody measurements, 72, 100
    vaccinations for, 70, 99
Membrane attack complex (MAC), 256, 285
Meningitis
    aseptic meningitis, 55, 85
    bacterial, 6, 126, 163
    diagnosis of, 114, 151
    H. influenzae, 143
    HSV meningitis, 53, 83
    treatment for, 30, 46
Methicillin-resistant *Staphylococcus aureus* (MRSA), 7, 31, 46, 122, 158
Microsporum species, 9, 192, 205
    M. audouini, 204
    M. canis, 190, 199, 200, 203–204, 210
Mitomycin, 21, 40
Mononucleosis, 51, 66, 67, 71, 81, 96–97, 99–101
Moraxella catarrhalis, 127, 163–164
Mucor, 10, 196, 208
Mumps virus, 4, 53, 69, 83, 93, 98
Mutations (genes), 30, 45

Mycobacterium species, 35, 47–48
    M. avium, 125, 161
    M. leprae, 7
    M. tuberculosis, 7, 127, 163
Mycology, 9–10
Mycoplasma species, 9, 173, 182
    M. hominis, 179, 187
    M. orale, 179, 187
    M. pneumoniae, 9, 109, 139, 145, 170, 179, 187
    M. salivarium, 187
    M. urealyticum, 9
Myeloperoxidase catalyzes, 2, 9

N

NADPH oxidase catalyzes, 9, 252, 284
Natural killer cells, 13, 258, 289
Neisseria species, 118, 154–155
    N. gonorrhoeae, 6, 17–18, 37–38, 111, 127, 147, 163
    N. menigitidis, 6, 34, 47–48, 139, 170
Norwalk virus, 75, 102, 103
Nucleic acid probes, 25, 42–43

O

Organisms, transfer of, 126–127, 163
Ornithosis, 174, 182
Orthomyxoviruses, 5, 77, 104–105
Ouchterlony gel diffusion test, 252, 283–284

P

Papillomavirus, 54, 61, 64, 71, 73, 76, 84, 91, 92, 93, 99, 101, 104
Parainfluenza viruses, 54, 84, 93
Paramyxoviruses, 4, 54, 78, 84, 93, 104–105
Parasites, 11–12
    diagnosis of, 229, 242
    raw fish consumption and, 218, 235
Parvovirus, 3, 49, 61, 80, 92
Pasteurella multocida, 7, 108, 133, 142, 145, 152, 166
Penicillin-binding proteins, 19, 39
Penicillins, 15, 36
    growth curves of, 26, 43
    spheroplasts of *E. coli*, 24, 42
    uses for, 129–130, 165
Periplasmic space, 16, 29, 36, 44
Peroxidase, 17, 36–37
Phialophora verrucosa, 198, 209

Plasmodium species, 11, 236
  P. falciparum, 216, 221, 223, 226, 234,
    236, 237, 239
Platelets, 247, 279
Pneumocystis, 224, 238
Pneumonia, 7
  C. pneumoniae, 8, 140, 171, 178, 186
  H. influenzae, 143
  L. pneumophila, 7, 113, 129, 140, 143,
    148–149, 165, 170–171
  M. pneumoniae, 9, 109, 139, 145, 170,
    179, 187
  pneumococcal pneumonia, 129, 165
  Pneumocystis carinii pneumonia (PCP),
    10, 197, 208, 224, 237
  S. aureus, 60, 90
  S. pneumoniae, 5, 7, 35, 48, 126, 150,
    162
Pneumonic plague, 123, 159
Poliovirus, 4, 91, 95
Polymerase chain reaction, 17–18, 23–24,
    25, 33–34, 37–38, 41–42, 43, 47
Polyomavirus, 77, 104
Precipitation reactions, 260, 290–291
Prions, 29, 44–45, 56, 59, 87, 90
Progressive multifocal leukoencephalopathy,
    77, 104
Pseudallescheria, 191, 204
Pseudomembranous enterocolitis, 130,
    165
Pseudomonads, 121, 157–158

Q
Q fever, 8, 128, 164, 173, 174, 181, 182,
    182–183
Quellung test, 126, 162

R
Rabies virus, 56, 57, 69, 87, 88, 98
Respiratory syncytial virus, 4, 58, 59, 69,
    89, 93, 98
Reverse transcriptase enzyme, 64, 93–94
Rhabdovirus, 5, 57, 88
Rheumatic fever (RF), 125, 161
Rh immunization, 267, 296
Rhinoviruses, 4, 56, 69, 87, 98
Rhizopus, 10, 196, 208, 211
Ribavirin, 52, 58, 82, 89
Rickettsiae species, 8, 173, 176, 182, 184
  R. akari, 176, 184
  R. prowazekii, 177, 178, 185, 186

Rickettsiae species (*Cont.*):
  R. rickettsii, 8, 177, 181, 182, 184, 185, 188
  R. tsutsugamushi, 177, 185
  R. typhi, 182
Ringworm, 9, 210
RNA viruses, 3, 4–5, 52, 82, 91
Rocky Mountain spotted fever, 8, 173, 175,
    176, 181, 182, 183, 184, 188
Rotaviruses, 5
  pediatric gastroenteritis, 62, 63, 74, 92, 93,
    102, 103
  vaccine for, 71, 99
Rubella virus, 4, 56, 59, 87, 90

S
Saint Louis encephalitis, 4, 64, 90, 94
Salmonella, 6, 18, 38–39
Sarcoptes scabiei, 226, 239–240
Schistosomiasis, 11, 227, 230, 240, 243
Scrapie, 44–45, 59, 90
Severe combined immunodeficiency syn-
    drome (SCID), 268, 294, 296
Shigella, 6, 127, 163
Shingles, 4, 83
Siderophores, 16, 36
Smallpox, 57, 88
Southern blot test, 24, 33, 42, 47
Spheroplasts, 2, 24, 42
Sporothrix schenckii, 10, 192, 198, 201, 205,
    209, 212
Sporozoans, 11
Spotted fever, 177, 185
  (*See also* Rocky Mountain spotted fever)
Sputum, 110, 146
Staphylococcus species, 158
  methicillin-resistant *S. aureus* (MRSA), 7,
    31, 46, 122, 158
  S. aureus, 2, 5, 15, 36, 60, 90, 108, 117,
    119, 142, 154, 156, 158
  S. epidermidis, 135, 158, 167
  S. saprophyticus, 158
Streptococcus species, 5, 34, 47–48
  antibiotics for, 130, 165
  group A streptococci, 124, 160
  group B streptococcal (GBS) disease,
    115–116, 151–152
  α-hemolytic streptococci, 135, 167–168
  Peptostreptococci, 5
  S. agalactiae, 5, 115–116, 150, 151–152
  S. bovis, 150
  S. faecalis, 5, 150

Streptococcus species (*Cont.*):
  S. *mutans*, 136, 168
  S. *pneumoniae*, 5, 7, 35, 48, 126, 150, 162
  S. *pyogenes*, 2, 5, 138, 150, 169–170
  S. *salivarius*, 136, 168
  S. *viridans*, 5, 125, 150, 161
Strongyloides, 12, 225, 229, 239, 242
Subacute sclerosing panencephalitis (SSPE),
  62, 93, 248, 263, 282, 294
Sulfonamides, 27, 43
Superoxide dismutase catalyzes, 2, 9, 16, 17,
  36–37
Syphilis, 112–113, 116, 148, 149, 152
Systemic lupus erythematosus (SLE), 14, 277,
  301

T
Taenia species
  T. *saginata*, 11, 218, 219, 234–235,
    235–236
  T. *solium*, 11, 218, 235
T cell lymphotrophic/leukemia virus (HTLV),
  91, 92
T cells, 13, 257, 269, 287, 296–297
Thayer-Martin (TM) agar, 133, 166
Thiosulfate citrate bile salts sucrose medium,
  134, 166
Tinea, 9
  tinea capitis, 9, 200, 210
  tinea corporis, 9, 197, 199, 208–209, 210
  tinea cruris, 9, 209
  tinea pedis, 9, 199, 210
  tinea versicolor, 200, 210
Toxic shock syndrome (TSS), 120, 156–157
Toxocara species, 231, 243
Toxoplasma species, 230, 243
  T. *encephalitis*, 220, 236
  T. *gondii*, 11, 100–101, 215, 219, 233, 235
Treponema pallidum, 7, 113, 148, 153
Trichinosis, 12, 230, 231, 243, 244
Trichomonas vaginalis, 11, 144, 224, 231, 238,
  243
Trichophyton, 9, 192, 205
Trypanosoma cruzi, 11, 221, 236
Tuberculosis, 110, 145
  M. *tuberculosis*, 7, 127, 163
Typhus, 177, 178, 185, 186

U
Ureaplasma urealyticum, 6, 174, 179, 183, 187

V
Vaccinations
  antibodies following, 249, 282–283
  Hepatitis A (HAV), 69, 99
  Hepatitis B (HBV), 70, 98
  immune status and, 248, 281
  influenza, 70, 98
  measles, 70, 99
  rabies virus, 69, 98
  rotaviruses, 71, 99
  secondary and booster, 259, 290
  smallpox, 57, 88
  types of, 14
Vaginitis, 108, 142, 144
Vancomycin-indeterminate *Staphylococcus
  aureus* (VISA), 7, 110, 146
Varicella-zoster virus, 4, 54, 73, 83–84, 101,
  293–294
Vibrio species, 7
  V. *cholerae*, 7, 106, 131, 142, 165
  V. *parahaemolyticus*, 7, 131, 165
  V. *vulnificus*, 7, 131, 166
Viruses, 3–5
  comparison to prions, 29, 44–45
  complement fixation antibody measure-
    ments, 72, 100
  disease patterns, 3
  growth cycles of, 3
  interferon and, 65, 95
  specimen collection for detection, 73–74,
    101
  terms for, 3

W
Western blot test, 22, 41, 255–256, 285
Western equine encephalitis, 4, 58, 88–89
West Nile virus, 4, 77, 104
Wiskott-Aldrich syndrome, 14, 264, 294
Wuchereria bancrofti, 12, 227, 241

X
Xenograft, 265, 294

Y
Yersinia species
  Y. *enterocolitica*, 132, 166
  Y. *pestis*, 7, 30, 46, 123, 152, 159

Z
Zygomycosis, 200, 201, 208